ABC OF ALLERGIES

ABC OF ALLERGIES

edited by

STEPHEN R DURHAM

*Reader and Honorary Consultant Physician, Upper Respiratory Medicine,
Imperial College School of Medicine, National Heart and Lung Institute
and Royal Brompton Hospital London, UK*

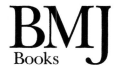

The image on the front cover is taken from a photograph of Dactylis glomerata (Cocksfoot grass) pollen grain taken at 3 500 magnification with a Scanning Electron Microscope. Courtesy of Dr Jean Emberlin National Pollen Research Unit, University College, Worcester.
Back cover image of house dust mites (background) with human skin (foreground) produced with permission from the Central Science Laboratory, York.

First published 1998
Second impression 1999
Third impression 2000
by BMJ Books, BMA House, Tavistock Square, London WC1H 9JR

British Library Cataloguing in Publication Data

A catalogue record for this book is avaialble from the British Library

ISBN 0-7279-1236-4

Typeset by Apek Typesetters, Nailsea, Bristol
Printed and bound by Craft Print, Singapore

Contents

Contributors

Carsten Bindslev-Jensen
Associate Professor, Department of Dematolgy, Aarhus Marseilisborg Hospital, Denmark

Sallie Buck
Practice Nurse, Exeter, Devon and Regional Trainer, National Asthma and Respiratory Training centre, Warwick.

Roger J Buckley
Consultant Ophthalmologist, Moorfields Eye Hospital, London, Professor of Ocular Medicine, City University, London

Peter Burney
Professor of Public Health Medicine, United Medical and Dental School, St Thomas' Hospital, London

Susan Cross
Director of Training, National Asthma and Respiratory Training Centre, Warwick

Paul Cullinan
Senior Lecturer, Occupational and Environmental Medicine, Imperial College School of Medicine, National Heart and Lung Institute, London

Adnan Custovic
Specialist Regristar in Allergy, North West Lung Centre, Wythenshawe Hospital, Manchester

Robert J Davies
Professor of Respiratory Medicine, Department of Asthma and Allergy, London Chest Hospital, London

Stephen R Durham
Reader and Honorary Consultant Physician, Upper Respiratory Medicine, Imperial College School of Medicine, National Heart and Lung Institute, and Royal Brompton Hospital, London

Pamela W Ewan
Medical Research Council Clinical Scientist and Honorary Consultant in Allergy and Clinical Immunology, Addenbrooke's Hospital, Cambridge

Peter S Friedmann
Professor of Dermatology, Southampton General Hospital, Southampton

Malcolm W Greaves
Head of Clinical Dermatology, St John's Institute of Dermatology, St Thomas' Hospital, London

Peter H Howarth
Senior Lecturer in Medicine, School of Medicine, Southampton General Hospital, Southampton

Jane Hubbard
Practice Nurse, Kingston, Surrey and Regional Trainer, National Asthma and Respiratory Training Centre, Warwick

D Jarvis
Senior Lecturer, Division of Public Health Medicine, United Medical and Dental Schools, St Thomas' Hospital, London

A B Kay
Professor of Allergy and Clinical Immunology, National Heart and Lung Institute, Imperial College School of Medicine, London

I S Mackay
Consultant ENT Surgeon, Royal Brompton Hospital and Charing Cross Hospital, London

A J Newman Taylor
Professor and Consultant Physician in Respiratory Medicine, Royal Brompton Hospital, London

Csaba Rusznak
Registrar in Respiratory Medicine and Allergy, Department of Asthma and Allergy, London Chest Hospital, London

Ruth A Sabroe
Honorary Senior Registrar, Professional Unit, St John's Institute of Dermatology, St. Thomas' Hospital, London

Daniel Vervloet
Professor of Chest Diseases, Allergy Division, Chest Diseases department, Hôpital Sainte Marguerite, Marseille, France

Ashley Woodcock
Consultant Respiratory Physician, North West Lung Centre, Wythenshawe Hospital, Manchester

Foreword

It is important to distinguish between atopy and allergy. Atopy refers to a tendency to develop exaggerated IgE responses to common inhaled allergens, and is manifested as a positive skin prick test and/or raised serum IgE to one or more common inhaled allergens, i.e. a predisposition to develop allergic diseases. Allergy, on the other hand, refers to the clinical expression of allergic disease and cannot be diagnosed by a skin prick test alone. Allergic diseases that are commonly associated with atopy include asthma, hayfever and eczema. These disorders are increasing in prevalence in developed countries.

The general practitioner, with the assistance of the practice nurse is quite rightly the first port of call for patients suffering from allergies. Unfortunately, allergy is not currently part of many undergraduate medical school curricula and there are limited resources for training in allergic disease at postgraduate level.

The *ABC of Allergies* provides guidelines for accurate diagnosis and management of common allergic disorders. Less common but important conditions such as venom allergy and anaphylaxis are also expertly covered. There is much practical advice on drug therapy, allergen avoidance measures and when to refer selected patients for allergen injection immunotherapy.

The chapter on "Good Allergy Practice" defines the resources required for an effective NHS allergy clinic at district general hospital level. The final chapter "Allergy in General Practice" identifies what can be achieved in partnership between the general practitioner and practice nurse and when to refer patients for specialist allergy advice.

Tak H Lee
National Asthma Campaign Professor
Department of Allergy and Respiratory Medicine
United Medical and Dental School, London
President, British Society for Allergy and Clinical Immunology

1 Good allergy practice

A B Kay

Allergic diseases result from an exaggerated response of the immune system to external substances. They are a common and increasing cause of illness and in Britain affect about 1 in 6 of the population. The annual cost to the NHS and the Department of Health for asthma alone is in excess of £750m. Although the public is concerned that the NHS has inadequate facilities for diagnosing and treating allergic diseases, there are many allergy clinics in the NHS. These are usually linked to specific specialties (such as chest diseases; ear, nose, and throat disease; paediatrics; dermatology; and gastroenterology). The British Society for Allergy and Clinical Immunology provides a regularly updated list of allergy clinics in the NHS (obtainable from the BSACI Secretariat, Membership Services, 66 Weston Park, Thames Ditton, Surrey, KT7 0HL).

Resources required

Allergy specialists

An overlap exists between allergology and other organ specialties. Hospital based allergy specialists in the NHS will usually be of consultant status and have appropriate training and experience. They will be either "physician immunologists"—trained in clinical immunology and allergy—or organ based specialists with an interest in allergy. In the future, specialist training will lead to a certificate of completion of specialist training in allergy. All health districts probably need at least one specialist in allergic diseases; if they do not have a consultant allergist or physician immunologist they should have an organ based specialist with an interest in allergy.

Outpatient facilities

Hospitals should have designated areas for both adult and paediatric allergy clinics organised by appropriately trained staff. Allergy consultations are often lengthy, and therefore a well organised appointments system is needed. The average consultation time for a new patient should be at least 30 minutes. For follow up visits no doctor should see more than four patients in an hour. Patients should be seen by, or have their cases discussed with, the consultant at the first visit and on regular occasions when follow up attendance is needed. Allergy clinics should provide opportunities for specialist training.

Facilities should be available for skin testing, spirometry (including peak flow measurements), supervising a patient's inhaler technique, providing asthma education and advice on avoiding allergens, instructing on self administration of adrenaline, and giving specific allergen injection immunotherapy (hyposensitisation) with an appropriate observation area. Allergen injection immunotherapy should be used routinely only in hay fever that is inadequately controlled by antiallergic drugs and in anaphylaxis resulting from hypersensitivity to wasp or bee venom; there must be immediate access to resuscitative facilities, and patients should be observed for 60 minutes (longer if even mild symptoms of hypersensitivity reactions develop).

Where appropriate, facilities should also be available for patients to have a chest x ray examination at the time of the clinic visit and for the radiographic film to be available for the consultation.

Most major hospitals have facilities for allergy testing

Good allergy practice

- Teamwork by doctors, nurses, and dietitians is essential
- The investigation of allergic diseases includes skin tests and challenge procedures—that is, tests for food allergy—as well as various specialised laboratory investigations
- Good clinical practice by providers and the effective use of allergy services by purchasers should improve prognosis and cut the costs of treating allergic diseases

---

Areas covered by allergy specialists

- Summer hay fever (seasonal, allergic, conjunctivorhinitis)
- Perennial rhinitis
- Allergic asthma (including occupational asthma)
- Allergy to stinging insects (especially wasps and bees)
- Allergy to drugs
- Allergy related skin disorders—namely, urticaria, angio-oedema, atopic eczema, and contact dermatitis
- Food allergy and intolerance
- Anaphylaxis

Summary of guidelines on specific allergen injection immunotherapy*

- Use only high quality standardised allergen extracts
- Administer in hospitals or specialised clinics only. Doctors should have appropriate experience and training in immunotherapy
- Adrenaline should always be immediately available
- Ready access to resuscitative facilities; attendant staff should be trained in resuscitative techniques
- Patients should be kept under close supervision for the first 60 minutes after each injection

*From the Royal College of Physicians and Royal College of Pathologists

ABC of Allergies

The support of an allergy clinic nurse is strongly recommended. Nurses with appropriate training can sometimes help in obtaining an allergy history. They can also perform skin tests and give advice on environmental control—for example, for minimising exposure to the house dust mite.

Qualified adult and paediatric dietitians should also be available, especially in clinics that deal with many cases of food allergy. They give detailed advice on exclusion diets—which commonly exclude peanuts, milk and milk products, fish, shellfish, egg, wheat and other foods as indicated by the history and investigations. Dietitians also assess the adequacy of diets that patients have used at their own or others' instigation—this may entail advising on the reintroduction of foods which either had been withdrawn from the diet with minimal indication of intolerance or may now be tolerated. Advice is also given on diets that reduce colorants, additives, or salicylates when indicated.

Special facilities at regional centres should include facilities for measuring non-specific bronchial hyper-responsiveness and challenge chambers for use with occupational agents (and occasionally common aeroallergens).

Skin prick tests

A diagnosis of allergy is based first on a careful clinical history. Skin tests should be used to support (or discount) a diagnosis of allergy. The skin prick test is the method of choice for diagnosing immediate-type (IgE mediated) hypersensitivity. In general, allergy testing by intradermal injection is not recommended, although it is sometimes used in diagnosing venom allergy. Skin test solutions must be standardised (biological standardisation is the most reliable) and should have a United Kingdom product licence. In Britain virtually all atopic subjects will give a positive reaction to an extract of one or more of the following: grass pollen, tree pollen, house dust mite, and cat and dog. These are the commonest allergens in allergic rhinitis and allergic asthma.

Other skin test solutions can be used less frequently—that is, when suggested by the clinical history. These include moulds (for example, alternaria or cladosporium), weeds, certain foods (for example, egg, milk, some nuts, fish and shellfish, where skin test solutions are known to have an established value), stinging insects (for example, bee and wasp venom), drugs (for example, penicillin derivatives, anaesthetic agents), and other animals (for example, horse, hamster).

Patch tests

Most cases of contact dermatitis are irritant dermatitis, but up to 40% are due to cell mediated allergic reactions, and the sensitising agent can be identified by patch testing. This procedure requires a comprehensive knowledge of the chemical allergens to which patients are exposed in specific work and leisure activities, as well as the nature of cross reacting chemicals. Interpreting allergic versus irritant reactions and appraising the significance of patch test results can be difficult even for clinicians experienced in this technique.

Dermatologists or allergists can best advise on avoidance and on the appropriate topical or systemic treatment.

Food allergy tests

Facilities should be available for open exclusion and reintroduction of food for allergy diagnosis as well as double blind, placebo controlled tests to identify or disprove food intolerance by giving suspected foods in disguised forms. For this purpose some pharmacies at specialist centres stock foodstuffs contained in special capsules, with placebo controls of similar appearance.

Role of specialist nurse in allergy clinic

- Skin testing
- Spirometry (including peak flow measurements)
- Supervision of a patient's inhaler technique
- Provision of asthma education
- Advice on the avoidance of allergens
- Instruction in self-administration of adrenaline
- Involvement in specific allergen injection immunotherapy (hyposensitisation)

Role of dietitian in allergy clinic

- Advice on exclusion diets
- Adequacy of diets
- Reintroduction of foods that have been withdrawn
- Advice on reducing colorants, additives, or salicylates when indicated

---

Performing a skin prick test

- A positive (histamine 10 mg/ml) and negative (diluent) control must always be included when performing skin prick tests (antihistamine drugs can blunt or inhibit the reactions)
- Ideally, antihistamines should be discontinued for 48 hours (long acting antihistamines for 21 days) before skin prick tests
- A positive reaction is usually regarded as being a weal ⩾2 mm greater than the negative control

---

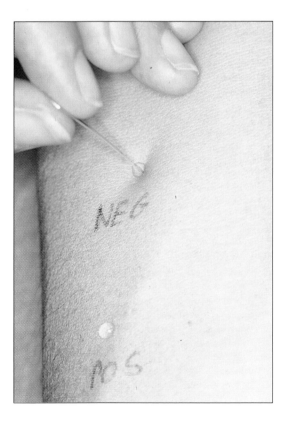

Skin prick testing showing positive and negative control

Laboratory investigations

Allergists should have access to routine haematology and biochemistry services as well as to certain immunological tests. If immunology tests cannot be done at an allergist's own hospital then samples should be sent to a regional immunology centre that has a consultant (or equivalent) immunologist and is accredited by Clinical Pathology Accreditation UK (the national accrediting body).

The most commonly used serological allergy tests are measurements of total and specific IgE antibodies to allergens relevant to the patient's symptoms. These tests are relatively expensive and are often unnecessary. They rarely give more information than skin tests, and so requests for such tests must be justified. They are useful in patients who have been taking antihistamines that suppress the skin test reaction; in patients with skin disease that is so extensive that skin tests are difficult to perform or who have dermatographism; when skin test results are equivocal or the patient has a history of anaphylaxis.

A positive specific IgE antibody test indicates a level of biological sensitivity to the relevant allergen, which may persist in the absence of symptoms. Therefore, as with skin tests, they must be interpreted in the context of the patient's history.

Other laboratory tests sometimes needed include immuno-chemical and functional measurements of the C1 esterase inhibitor for diagnosing hereditary and acquired angio-oedema; IgG antibodies (for example, precipitin tests) to fungal and avian products and other relevant material for use in diagnosing extrinsic allergic alveolitis. Very occasionally, specialist tests may be appropriate—for example, lymphocyte transformation for drug and venom allergy, and measurements of urinary and plasma mediators such as histamine and tryptase in the differential diagnosis of anaphylaxis.

Paediatric allergy

Allergic diseases are particularly important in children, and paediatricians should always participate in the diagnosis and management of children referred for specialist care. However, although paediatricians study allergy in their general training, they may decide to consult with, or refer a child to, an adult allergy specialist. The progression of allergies in children differs from that in adults—for example, food allergies and insect venom anaphylaxis. Drug treatments are different for children both in dosage and side effects. The inherent dangers of unnecessary dietary restriction for treating some types of allergic diseases are far greater in children because of disturbances in nutrition and growth, and expert paediatric dietetic advice is usually required. Techniques for cardiopulmonary resuscitation after anaphylaxis are not the same as those in adults.

There seems to be widespread public misunderstanding about the contribution of allergies to diverse children's diseases, such as hyperactivity, other forms of behavioural disorder, recurrent abdominal pain, and chronic headaches. Such children must be seen by paediatricians within the framework of a comprehensive children's department.

The illustration of allergenic foods was prepared by Jan Croot.

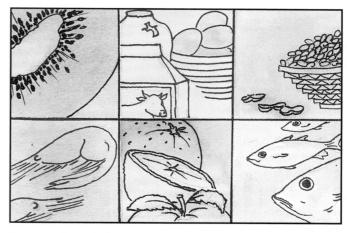

Common allergenic foods

Patients with allergy and the role of alternative practitioners*

More trials needed in
- Homoeopathy
- Acupuncture
- Hypnosis
- Enzyme potentiated desensitisation (enzyme digested substances injected into the skin)

Not recommended
- Tests used by clinical ecologists or "environmentalists"—neutralisation-provocation (Miller) test and neutralisation vaccines (based on multiple skin tests to foods and environmental agents such as smoke, petrol, and tobacco)
- Leucocytotoxic tests
- Hair analysis
- Vega testing (a "black box" electrical test)
- Applied kinesiology (allergy tests based on "muscle weakness")
- Auricular cardiac reflex testing (allergy tests based on the pulse rate)
- Treatments based on the "candida hypersensitivity syndrome" and "allergy" to mercury or dental amalgam

*According to Royal College of Physicians

What is a good allergy clinic? Guidance for purchasers

- The person in charge of an allergy clinic should be of consultant status and have had approved higher medical training in a field related to allergy
- There should be adequate support staff, which would normally include an allergy clinic nurse and access to a qualified dietitian
- There should be facilities for skin testing and access to an approved laboratory for investigations such as measurements of specific IgE antibodies and other immunological tests as appropriate
- Allergy clinics that offer allergen injection immunotherapy should follow recommended guidelines
- Allergy clinics should use methods of diagnosis and treatment of proved efficacy

---

This article is based on the report *Good Allergy Practice—Standards of Care for Providers and Purchasers of Allergy Services within the National Health Service* by the Royal College of Physicians and the Royal College of Pathologists, reproduced in *Clinical and Experimental Allergy* and edited by Professor A B Kay.

2 The epidemiology of allergic disease

D Jarvis, P Burney

Atopy is defined as the production of specific IgE in response to exposure to common environmental allergens, such as house dust mite, grass, and cat. Being atopic is strongly associated with allergic disease such as asthma, hay fever, and eczema, but not everyone with atopy develops clinical manifestations of allergy and not everyone with a clinical syndrome compatible with allergic disease can be shown to be atopic when tested for specific IgE to a wide range of environmental allergens. This is particularly so for asthma.

Asthma is arguably the most serious of the allergic diseases in that it is disabling (causing more than 100 000 hospital admissions each year in England and Wales) and occasionally fatal. In 1995, 137 people aged under 45 died as a result of asthma. Although concern has been expressed that death certificates may overestimate or underestimate asthma mortality depending on diagnostic fashion, significant mis-classification with other forms of chronic obstructive lung disease in this age group is unlikely. In the early 1960s asthma mortality increased dramatically in many countries. The increase was attributed to the excessive use of non-selective β agonists, which were subsequently withdrawn from the market. More recent increases in asthma mortality reported from Britain, France, and the United States may be related to increased prevalence or severity of asthma or inadequate health care. Evidence for the latter comes from audits and confidential inquiries that show inadequate treatment of asthma in the months leading up to death and during the fatal attack and the observation of higher mortality in populations recognised as often receiving poor health care (socioeconomically deprived people in Britain; black people in the United States). In England and Wales asthma mortality rose between the mid-1970s and the mid-1980s but declined steadily during the early 1990s.

Hay fever and eczema are important causes of morbidity, being responsible for a substantial proportion of health service use, particularly in primary care, and reduced quality of life.

Prevalence

Time trends

The prevalence of diseases associated with atopy has increased in many parts of the world over the past 20 to 30 years. In the United Kingdom the prevalence of diagnosed asthma and symptoms strongly suggestive of asthma in children has increased at a rate of about 5% a year. Increases of a similar magnitude have been observed in Sweden, Switzerland, Norway, the United States, Australia, New Zealand, and Taipei. Some of this apparent rise may have occurred in response to greater public awareness of asthma and a greater tendency of parents to report wheezing illnesses in their children and to attend their doctor for treatment of asthma.

Few serial surveys have examined an increase in objective markers for asthma, although the prevalence of exercise induced bronchial constriction has increased in Welsh school-children over 15 years, suggesting that the increase in reported symptoms reflects a genuine change in health status. Few reported serial surveys have examined the prevalence of asthma in adults, although the proportion of military recruits with asthma has increased in Finland, Sweden, and Israel.

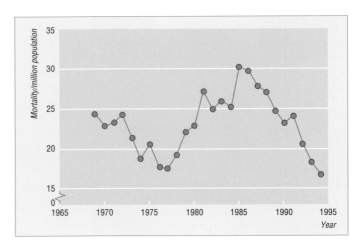

Age standardised asthma mortality, England and Wales, 1969–94 (both sexes, 15–64 years

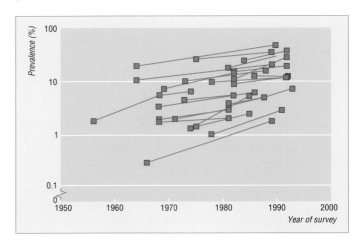

Changes in prevalence of asthma and wheeze, according to surveys conducted 1956–93 worldwide

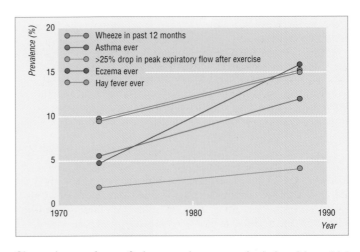

Change in prevalence of wheeze, asthma, excercise induced bronchial constriction, hay fever, and eczema in children in South Wales between 1973 and 1988

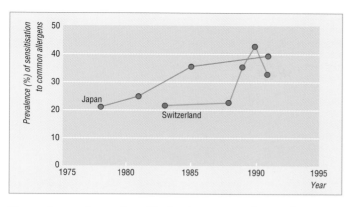

Change in prevalence of sensitisation to common allergens in schoolchildren in Japan and switzerland

Most of the surveys that have shown increases in the prevalence of asthma have also shown increases in the prevalence of other allergic diseases, such as hay fever and eczema. In the United Kingdom, results from the three national birth cohorts (samples of people born in 1946, 1958, and 1970) have shown a marked increase (5.1%, 7.3%, and 12.2% respectively) in the prevalence of eczema as reported by the mother in children aged under 5.

The rising prevalence of allergic disease has resulted in increased use of health services. For asthma, hospital admissions (particularly among children aged under 5 years), consultation with general practitioners, and the use of drug treatment all rose sharply during the 1980s. Consultations with general practitioners for managing hay fever also increased.

The increased prevalence of all allergic diseases suggests that the prevalence of atopy has increased. Epidemiological information from Switzerland and Japan shows that the prevalence of atopy is increasing in children. In both these studies the increase in the prevalence of atopy was due to an increase in sensitisation to a variety of allergens and not dominated by an increase in sensitisation to one particular allergen. In Britain no evidence exists that exposure to allergen has increased—in fact grass pollen levels have steadily decreased over the past 20 years and pet ownership has probably not changed. At present the extent to which changes in the prevalence of atopy and changes in allergen exposure explain the time trends in allergic disease is unknown.

Geographical distribution

Until recently the methods used for assessing the prevalence of allergic disease were not standardised and comparisons of disease prevalence between countries were flawed. Two major research initiatives, the European Community respiratory health survey (ECRHS) and the international study of asthma and allergies in childhood (ISAAC) have developed and executed standardised protocols for the assessment of disease prevalence in many different countries in adults and children.

The European Community respiratory health survey has shown wide geographical variation in the reported prevalence of symptoms highly suggestive of asthma, treatment for asthma, and current hay fever or nasal allergies in adults. In general, symptoms are more common in New Zealand, Australia, the British Isles, and the United States than in mainland Europe, although there is wide variation even within some countries. The distribution of atopy (for these purposes defined as sensitisation to house dust mite, grass, cat, or cladosporium species) shows a similar distribution, with marked variation between countries, although the extent to which variation in atopy explains variation in symptoms is still under investigation.

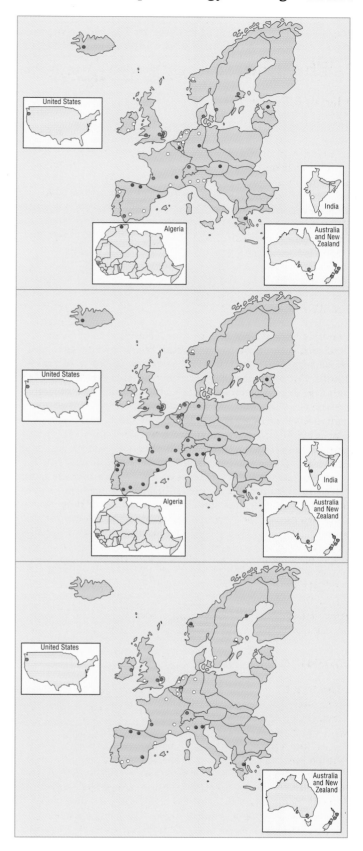

Areas with high (red) and (blue) prevalence of asthma (top), hay fever and nasal allergies (centre), and sensitisation to any one of house dust mite, cat, timothy grass, or cladosporium species (bottom), according to results of the European Community respiratory health survey (white circles represent areas that participated in the study but which did not have a particularly high or low prevalence

Prevalence (percentage) of self reported asthma symptoms in past year in children aged 12–15 years in five centres participating in the international study of asthma and allergies in childhood

	Bochum, Germany	West Sussex, UK	Wellington, New Zealand	Adelaide, Australia	Sydney, Australia
Sample size	1928	2097	1863	1428	1519
Wheeze in past year	20	29	28	29	30
Severe attack of wheezing in past year	6	7	11	10	13

The international study of asthma and allergies in childhood, which has not yet been fully reported, has shown that severe asthma is more common in children living in New Zealand and Australia than in those living in West Sussex and in Bochum, Germany.

Risk factors

Genetics
Total IgE concentration, the production of specific IgE, and bronchial hyperreactivity are all under some degree of genetic control. Chromosome 5 has been implicated in the regulation of total IgE concentration, chromosome 11q linked to the atopic phenotype (high total IgE concentration or specific IgE to a common allergen), and chromosome 14 linked to eczema; specific HLA haplotypes are linked to the development of IgE to some allergens (for example, specific allergens from rye grass are associated with DR3). Although genetic susceptibility to allergic disease is important, it is unlikely that either the large geographical variations in disease prevalence between peoples of similar genetic background, or the increase in allergic disease over the past few decades can be explained by genetic factors.

Age and sex
The incidence of asthma is higher in children than in adults. Longitudinal surveys suggest that children with mild disease are likely to become asymptomatic as teenagers, whereas those with more severe disease will have symptoms that persist throughout life. To some extent this "ageing" effect explains why in some cross sectional studies allergic disease is less common in adults than in children, but these observations may also reflect an increased propensity for asthma and atopy in those born later in the century.

More boys than girls have atopy, asthma, and hay fever, although these differences become less apparent later in life. At all ages, males have higher total IgE concentration than females.

Infection
More than 80% of asthma exacerbations in children are of viral origin. This epidemiological observation equates well with most clinical experience, but consensus is weaker over the role of infection in the pathogenesis of atopy and allergic disease.

Children who grow up in large families, especially if exposed to older siblings, are likely to experience more childhood infections than those who come from small families. Because the prevalence of allergic disease, in particular hay fever, and sensitisation to common allergens is lower in those who grow up in large families or who have older siblings, high rates of infection in childhood may protect against the development of atopy and allergic disease.

Secular changes in family structure and maternal smoking do not fully explain the increase in wheezing, hay fever, or eczema in adolescents.

Smoking
- People who smoke have higher total IgE concentration and are more likely to become sensitised to allergens in the workplace than people who do not.
- The association between smoking and sensitisation to common allergens, however, is not clear, with several reports of lower rates of sensitisation to common environmental allergens and less hay fever in smokers
- This may be explained to some extent by the 'healthy smoker' bias (the tendency of those with allergic disease not to smoke) but may also reflect a genuinely reduced incidence of some forms of allergy among smokers
- Smoking is an important risk factor for bronchial hyperreactivity—a feature of asthma—buts its association with asthma remains uncertain
- Children whose mothers smoke during pregnancy have reduced lung function and more wheezing illness during childhood but do not seem to have more allergic diseases

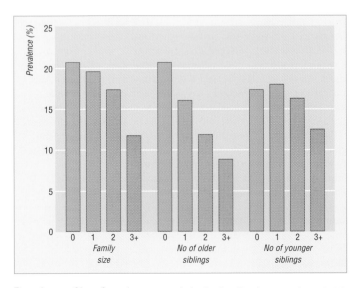

Prevalence of hay fever in young adults by family size, number of older siblings, and number of younger siblings

Exposure to allergens

The development of sensitisation to an allergen requires exposure to that allergen. Exposure early in life may be associated with a higher risk of sensitisation than exposure later in life, but no evidence exists yet that reducing allergen load in the home of young children reduces sensitisation or the development of allergic disease.

Once sensitisation has occurred, repeated exposure to that allergen is likely to trigger symptoms. Epidemics of asthma have occurred when high levels of allergen have been present in ambient air. In Barcelona outbreaks of asthma identified through sudden increases in emergency admissions for asthma resulted from unloading of soy beans at the local harbour. The epidemics were prevented by reducing the ambient allergen load by installing filters at the top of the storing tower. In Britain a severe thunderstorm in 1994 was associated with the largest ever outbreak of asthma. Many of the epidemic cases had previously experienced only hay fever, and asthma was probably precipitated in these grass sensitised individuals by the release during the thunderstorm of small aerosolised particles of grass allergen from grass pollen in the air. In Britain more deaths from asthma occur during the summer and early autumn than during the winter. This seasonal pattern is not observed in deaths from asthma in elderly people and may be another manifestation of the importance of allergens on the severity of asthma, particularly in young people.

In Britain most people with allergic disease are sensitised to house dust mite, and this allergen has been implicated as the most important allergen for both the development and exacerbation of asthma and eczema. In other countries sensitisation to cat, grass, or moulds may be a more important cause of disease.

More than 300 agents have been identified as occupational allergens. Occupational exposure to allergens may cause eczema, rhinitis, or asthma. Occupational exposure to agents known to cause asthma may be responsible for as many as 1 in 15 cases of adult onset asthma in some populations.

Diet

Over the past 20 years diet has dramatically altered in most developed countries. Sensitivity to food, particularly to milk, eggs, and fish, is not uncommon in childhood; in adults, though "intolerance to foodstuffs" is frequently reported, it is rarely observed on formal challenge. Withdrawal of allergenic foods may reduce the severity of some allergic disease. Other dietary factors such as electrolytes (sodium and magnesium), nature of fatty acids in the diet (in particular oily fish), and antioxidants have all been identified as possibly increasing the severity of asthma.

The data in the third graph are from Burr et al (*Arch Dis Child* 1989;64:1452-6); in the fourth graph are from Nakagomi et al (*Lancet* 1994;343:122-3) and Gassner et al (*Schweiz Rundschau Med* 1992;81:426-8); in the fifth graph are from Strachan D (*Clin Exp Allergy* 1995;25:296-303); and in the second table are from Meredith S (*J Epidemiol Community Health* 1993;47:459-63). The first table and the final graph are adapted with permission from Pearce et al (*Eur Respir J* 1993;1455-61) and the Office for National Statistics' *Health of Adult Britain*, respectively.

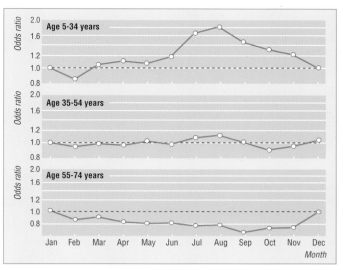

Odds of dying from asthma by month compared with odds of dying in January (England and Wales, 1958–91)

Incidence (95% confidence interval) of occupational asthma (cases per million workers per year) in some high risk occupational groups

Occupational group	Incidence
Coach and other spray painters	658 (508 to 839)
Chemical processors	364 (274 to 475)
Plastics workers	337 (248 to 448)
Bakers	334 (248 to 440)
Laboratory technicians and assistants	188 (139 to 247)
Workers in welding, soldering, and electronic assembly	175 (138 to 218)

Further reading

- European Community Respiratory Health Survey. Variations in the prevalence of respiratory symptoms, self-reported asthma attacks and the use of asthma medication in the European Community respiratory health survey (ECRHS). *Eur Respir J* 1996;9:687-95
- Burney P, Malmberg E, Chinn S, Jarvis D, Luczynska C, Lai E. The distribution of total and specific serum IgE in the European community respiratory health survey. *J Allergy Clin Immunol* 1997;99:314-22
- Barbee R, Kaltenbourn W, Lebowitz M, Burrows B. Longitudinal changes in allergen skin test reactivity in a community population sample. *J Allerg Clin Immunol* 1987;79:16-24
- Central Health Monitoring Unit. *Asthma: an epidemiological overview.* London: HMSO, 1995
- Burr M, ed. *Epidemiology of clinical allergy. Monographs in Allergy.* Vol 31. Basle: Karger, 1993

3 Diagnosing allergy

Csaba Rusznak, Robert J Davies

Allergy to environmental agents can affect almost every organ of the body. Although allergic rhinitis is the commonest manifestation, the lower respiratory tract, the conjunctiva, the skin, and the gastrointestinal tract are frequently affected by allergic disease.

Allergic diseases are common, and their prevalence is increasing. Accurate diagnosis of triggering or causative allergens is essential for appropriate advice for avoidance and environmental control measures. Although allergic diseases can occur at almost any age, some allergies are most likely to develop for the first time in particular age groups.

Symptoms

An immediate relation between exposure to potential allergens and the development of symptoms makes both the diagnosis and identification of allergy straightforward. In 25-50% of cases the predominant symptoms develop 1-10 hours after exposure (late phase reactions), obscuring the allergic nature of the illness. In allergic diseases of occupational aetiology the first symptom may be exercise induced asthma or night-time waking with cough. The longer such symptoms have been present the more likely they are to persist when exposure ceases.

The onset of seasonal symptoms occurs three weeks earlier in southern England than in northern Scotland.

Symptoms occur more rapidly after exposure to the causative agent as sensitisation increases. Many patients with food allergy develop an intense dislike of the offending food. Symptoms are usually gastrointestinal (abdominal pain, bloating, vomiting, diarrhoea) or cutaneous (itching, urticaria, angio-oedema)—symptoms are less commonly respiratory (asthma) and are rarely related to rhinitis.

Cross reaction can occur between various allergens, such as birch tree pollen and certain foods (for example, apple, carrot, celery, potato, orange, tomato, hazelnut, and peanut). Cross reactivity also exists between latex and some fruits (banana, avocado, kiwi fruit, and chestnut).

Itching of the throat and ears is a common manifestation of pollen allergy, and patients allergic to house dust mite experience exacerbations when bedmaking, vacuum cleaning, and sleeping in damp accommodation.

The impact of the allergic symptoms on an individual's lifestyle should be assessed in terms of impairment of school or work performance and time missed, with particular emphasis on the interference in leisure activities and sleep.

Factors influencing development of allergic diseases

If both parents are allergic the risk of allergy in the offspring is 75%; if one parent is allergic the risk is 50%. The risk in the population is 10-20%. Allergy is much less common in younger children in large families than in their older siblings. This is probably due to viral infections being passed more often from one child to another in large families, which may influence the subsequent dominance of Th1 driven rather than Th2 driven immune responses.

Age when certain allergies are likely to occur for first time
- Infancy—Atopic dermatitis, food allergies (milk, egg, nuts)
- Childhood—Asthma (house dust mite, pets)
- Teenagers—Allergic rhinitis (grass and tree pollens)
- Early adulthod—Urticaria, angio-oedema (aspirin intolerance)
- Adulthood—Allergy to venom (bee, wasp)

Taking a clinical history
- A detailed clinical history is vital for diagnosing an allergy
- Taking a history requires experience, time, and patience
- Patients should be allowed to give their own account of their symptoms in their own time
- Structured questions about the patients' history (with particular emphasis on previous allergic diseases—such as childhood eczema, hay fever, and asthma) should be asked
- Frequency, severity, duration, and seasonality of symptoms should be ascertained, with particular reference to triggering factors, life threatening events, and effects of avoidance measures
- Patients should be asked about diet; food exclusion; and intolerance to aspirin, colourings, and preservatives
- Family history should be explored
- Home, work, and outdoor environmental risk factors should be discussed
- Groups at particular risk of allergy—such as healthcare and rubber industry workers and children with spina bifida, in whom latex allergy is particularly prevalent—should be identified
- Patients should be asked about any treatment they are currently using, particularly about antihistamines, topical and oral corticosteroids, and adrenalin autoinjectors

---

Environmental factors predisposing to development and triggering of allergy

Indoor
Damp and poorly ventilated dwelling
Old mattresses (not vacuumed or covered)
Unwashed and uncovered pillows and duvet
Pets
Cigarette smoke
Gas fired cooking stoves, boilers, and fires (not adequately ventilated to the outside)

Outdoor
Density of grains of grass or tree pollen in local environment
Presence of new aeroallergens—eg *Parietaria judaiica* (the wall pellitory) in southern England
Proximity to major roadways or power stations

Occupational
Isocyanate
Flour
Laboratory animals
Resin
Wood dust
Glutaraldehyde
Biological enzymes
Latex

Allergy tests in vivo

Skin tests

Skin prick test

The skin prick test is the most widely used allergy test and can be performed during the initial consultation with aqueous solutions of a variety of allergens. These include *(a)* common inhaled allergens (house dust mite, grass pollen, cat dander, dog hair); *(b)* occupational allergens (such as ammonium persulphate, platinum salts, antibiotics, and latex); and *(c)* food allergens.

Skin prick testing requires control using diluent (negative control) and histamine solution (positive control). A drop of allergen solution is placed on the skin of the forearm. A sterile lancet or 25 gauge (orange) needle is used to prick the skin through the allergen solution (a separate needle is used for each allergen solution). The excess allergen solution is removed from the skin with an absorbent paper tissue. The reaction is evaluated after 15 minutes.

The test should be performed with standardised allergen solutions, if possible. In general practice it may be sufficient to use four allergens (house dust mite, grass pollen, and cat and dog allergen) plus the positive and negative controls to confirm or exclude atopy and recognise the most common allergens encountered.

Test solutions are available from ALK Abello (Reading, Berkshire) under the brand name Soluprick.

A positive result is a skin weal > 2 mm greater than that observed with the negative control (allergen diluent) solution. However, the relation between a positive result and overt clinical disease caused by that allergen is not absolute. The concentration of the allergen solution will determine the result of the test. Ideally the test should combine the highest possible sensitivity with the highest possible specificity, but this degree of precision is not usually achievable.

The result of the skin prick test should be interpreted in the light of the clinical history: if both the history of allergy and the test result are positive, atopy and the offending allergen are confirmed; if both are negative, allergy is excluded; in the case of perennial allergens, there may not be an immediate association between exposure and symptoms, resulting in a false negative history in the context of a positive test result; many patients with a positive test result do not have symptoms of allergy; if there is discordance between the history and the test result, referral to an allergy specialist is recommended.

The advantages of skin prick testing are: it is painless and has a low risk of side effects; it is informative to the patient; patient compliance is high; and the test can be performed in health centres.

The disadvantages are: systemic and topical antihistamines may suppress the weal and flare reaction; the test is less reliable with food allergens (which are less well standardised) than with inhaled allergens; itching causes a slight discomfort; and interpretation is difficult in patients with eczema or dermatographism.

Although skin prick testing with inhaled allergens is generally safe, occasional systemic reactions including anaphylaxis have been reported when food allergens are used; testing with food allergens should therefore be performed only in specialist centres. Adrenaline should always be available.

Intracutaneous test

The intracutaneous test is rarely indicated, though it is of value in the diagnosis of drug or venom allergy.

It should be performed by allergy specialists in specialist centres.

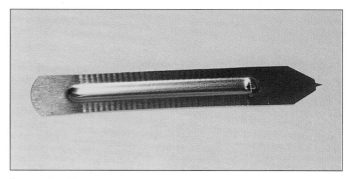

Lancet for skin prick testing

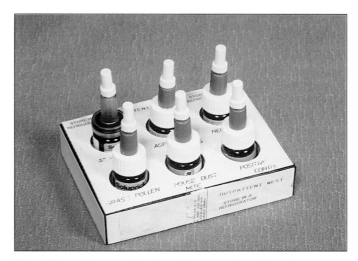

Skin prick test kit comprising four allergens and positive control solution (histamine 10 mg/ml) and negative control (allergen diluent)

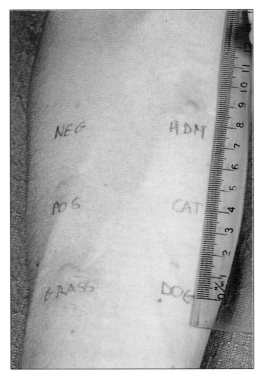

Evaluation at 15 minutes of skin prick test results (weal sizes in mm)

ABC of Allergies

Patch test

The patch test is widely used in the diagnosis of allergic contact dermatitis. Several standardised series of contact allergens are available. Possible allergens are applied in a standardised form to a healthy area of the patient's skin. The patch test can be performed either with the suspected chemicals or with the standard series of allergens.

Eczematous reaction at the site of application 48-72 hours later shows that the patient is sensitised to that allergen. The reaction must be distinguished from simple irritant reactions.

The patch test is the most important diagnostic tool in diagnosing contact allergic dermatitis. However, patch testing can cause a flare up reaction (of healed eczema) or persisting test reactions. It can also cause sensitisation and subsequent allergic contact dermatitis. It is time consuming, and it requires specialist interpretation.

Bronchial, nasal, and conjunctival provocation tests

These tests are rarely required in the routine diagnosis of allergy. Bronchial or nasal provocation test with allergen may occasionally be useful in determining "local sensitisation," in which, although the results of skin prick testing (and of the radioallergosorbent test, if also done) are negative, the airways are responsive to the specific allergen. These tests must be performed only by individuals trained in allergy diagnosis.

Food challenge

Diagnosis of food allergy requires taking a careful history and, if necessary, altering the patient's diet with the help of a skilled dietician. The consequence of correct diagnosis can be beneficial to patients but may disrupt their lifestyle. A definite diagnosis of food allergy can be established by properly conducted blinded food challenges, which avoid any possible bias from patient or investigator.

Food challenge will be covered in more detail in a later chapter on food allergy.

Common examples of contact allergy

Agent	Source
Mercury	Topical ointments
Cobalt	Metal plated objects, wet cement
Fragrance	Cosmetics, household chemicals
Nickel	Coins, alloys, insecticides
p-Phenylenediamine	Hair dye, fur dye
Paraben	Cosmetics
Imidazolidinyl urea	Cosmetics (preservatives)
Formalin, formaldehyde	Cosmetics, insecticides
Carba mix	Rubber, fungicides
Thiuram	Rubber compounds, fungicides
Epoxy resin	Adhesives

Food challenge

- Removal of the food from the patient's diet should eliminate symptoms
- Ideally challenges should be conducted as double blind, placebo controlled challenges
- If the suspected food, but not the inactive substance, causes an allergic reaction, the diagnosis is established
- Food challenges must be performed under strict medical supervision and in hospital settings
- Food challenges, however, may cause anaphylactic reaction, are time consuming, and require several challenges, with washout periods of days

Allergy tests in vitro

Nasal smears

Nasal smear tests are used to determine the number of eosinophils present in the nasal secretion. A cotton bud is inserted two or three times into each nostril, and the lining of the nose scraped with a firm, rolling movement. Secretions are spread gently on to a microscope slide and stained, and the cells are counted.

The advantages of nasal smears are that the nose is readily accessible and the test can help to differentiate between eosinophilic rhinitis (allergic rhinitis and non-allergic rhinitis with eosinophilia, which respond well to topical corticosteroids) and rhinitis due to other causes. However, the disadvantages are a slight discomfort to the patient and a high risk of false negative results if the nasal smear is not properly obtained.

If more than 10% of the stained cells in nasal smears are eosinophils this indicates a positive result compatible with nasal eosinophilia

Serum allergen specific IgE concentrations

In the radioallergosorbent test (RAST) allergens (antigens) are chemically bound to an insoluble matrix such as plastic, cellulose nitrate, cellulose (paper), or agarose beads. When patients' serum is added, allergen specific IgE binds to immobilised allergen. Radioactively labelled anti-IgE is then added, which attaches to the specific IgE already bound to the allergen. The amount of specific IgE in the patient's blood can be estimated from the amount of bound radioactivity.

In another type of allergosorbent test (the CAP-RAST system) the allergen is covalently coupled to a cellulose carrier

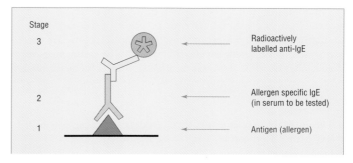

The principle of the radioallergosorbent test

10

with a large surface area. The patient's serum containing IgE is then added and specific IgE reacts with bound allergen. After non-specific IgE has been washed away, enzyme labelled antibodies against human IgE are added, and the bound complex is then incubated with a fluorescence substrate, the developing agent.

An enzyme linked immunosorbent assay (ELISA) is a non-radioactive method which uses antigen in fluid phase and enzyme labelling of anti-IgE, which is detected by adding substrate for the enzyme, which produces colour change detected photometrically.

The radioactivity (radioallergosorbent test), fluorescence (CAP-RAST test), or colour (enzyme linked immunosorbent assay) of the eluate corresponds with the concentration of specific IgE in the patient's blood.

The advantages of measuring the concentration of allergen specific IgE are that (a) it is not influenced by any concurrent drug treatment, (b) it can be performed when there is widespread skin disease, (c) it is completely safe, (d) the specificity of the two radioallergosorbent tests can be as high as 90% for inhaled allergens. However, the results are not immediately available, and testing is expensive.

Alternative tests

- Recently there has been a surge in the number of alternative "allergy tests" offered direct to patients—for example, the antigen leucocyte cellular antibody test, hair analysis, bioresonance diagnostics, autohomologous immune therapy, electroacupuncture, and vega testing
- No scientific evidence exists that these tests are useful in diagnosing allergy
- Such tests may also disadvantage patients, who may modify diet and lifestyle to no avail

4 Pathogenic mechanisms: a rational basis for treatment

Peter H Howarth

Allergic diseases such as asthma, rhinitis, eczema, and anaphylaxis are increasingly common and, in addition to being associated with morbidity and potential mortality, constitute a considerable burden on health resources, with both direct and indirect costs. This article discusses the pathogenic mechanism underlying the clinical signs and symptoms of these diseases and explains the basis for the choice of differing treatments.

Relation of atopy and allergy to disease

About 40% of the population is atopic as evidenced by a positive response to a skin prick test with an allergen, but not all show signs and symptoms of clinical disease. There may be a latency period, as students who have positive skin prick tests with grass pollen but who do not experience hay fever have been shown to go on to develop seasonal allergic rhinitis. A threshold response may also be required for signs and symptoms of clinical disease to develop, as allergic airway inflammation is present in the lower airways of patients with perennial allergic rhinitis sensitive to house dust mite who do not have clinical asthma. This inflammatory response falls between the response in patients with clinical asthma and that in non-atopic healthy controls.

The situation is, however, more complex than this, as patients with comparable responses to skin prick testing may have solely asthma, rhinitis, or eczema, and current research to explain organ-specific disease is focusing on the local tissue production of IgE and on the role of selective homing and activation of T lymphocytes, which may amplify the local tissue response. It is, however, possible in sensitised individuals to link allergen exposure to signs and symptoms of clinical disease, as seasonal exposure to aeroallergens (such as tree or grass pollens or fungal spores) induces seasonal allergic rhinoconjunctivitis, and exposure to perennial allergens (usually indoor allergens such as house dust mite or other animal allergens) is associated with persistent signs and symptoms of disease (asthma or rhinitis, or both). Intermittent exposure to systemic allergens, such as food, drugs, or venom, can induce acute disease (anaphylaxis, urticaria, dermatitis, asthma, rhinitis), which may take a variable time to resolve. IgE mediated reactions underlie these clinical responses.

Immunoglobulin E

An increase in specific IgE is reflected by positive skin prick tests to allergens or by positive in vitro tests such as the radioallergosorbent test. Specific IgE is generated by B lymphocytes under the regulation of cytokines generated by T lymphocytes. Cytokines are small molecular weight chemicals that have a localised action in modulating cell function. The cytokines that favour IgE isotype switching (interleukin 4 and interleukin 13) are generated by a subpopulation of T lymphocytes with a T helper 2 cytokine profile, whereas T cells that generate a T helper 1 cytokine profile—by secreting interferon gamma—inhibit B cell isotype switching for IgE synthesis. Th1 and Th2 cells reciprocally inhibit each other's development. In atopy the production of IgE is increased,

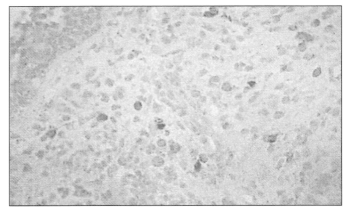
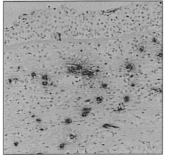
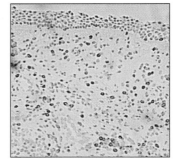

Immunohistology of nasal mucosa in allergic rhinitis using alkaline phosphatase/anti-alkaline phosphatase technique showing individual cells stained red: mast cells (top), eosinophils (bottom left), and CD4 T lymphocytes (bottom right)

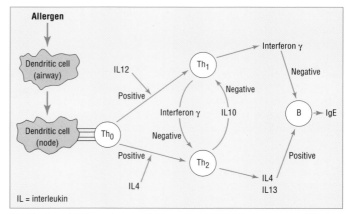

Regulation of B lymphocyte IgE synthesis by T lymphocytes. T cells with the Th2 cytokine profile increase interleukin 4 and interleukin 13 synthesis, which promotes IgE isotype switching, whereas the development of T cells with a Th1 cytokine profile, which generate the interferon gamma, inhibits B cell isotype switching for IgE synthesis. This process also involves antigen uptake and processing by mucosal dendritic cells (commonly Langerhans' cells in the airways) and the presentation of antigen in a modified format to T lymphocytes, typically in a draining lymph node

suggesting an imbalance in the ratio of Th2 to Th1 control. The development of Th2 secreting lymphocytes requires interleukin 4. This cytokine is generated by the placenta to prevent immunological fetal rejection (a Th1 cytokine response). It has been proposed that that persistence of this placental Th2 drive—possibly related to improved or altered nutrition in the absence of a Th1 counter switch—is the major factor contributing to the increasing prevalence of allergic disease in the past 30-40 years. An additional contributory factor may be a decrease in severe infection in early infancy over the same period and an interaction between allergens and atmospheric pollution that potentiates the tendency to sensitisation. Infection would drive a Th1 response and thus down regulate the tendency for Th2 related disease to develop.

Mediators of hypersensitivity

IgE binds to tissue mast cells and circulating basophils through cell-surface expressed high affinity receptors. Allergen binds to specific IgE and induces cell activation, with the tissue release and generation of mediators such as histamine, tryptase, leukotrienes, prostaglandins, and kinins from mast cells contributing to symptoms of asthma and rhinitis through direct actions on neural and vascular receptors and within the lower airways also on airway smooth muscle receptors.

Histamine and leukotriene release from basophils, as well as mediator release from mast cells, will contribute to circulatory events in anaphylaxis. The release of these mediators is rapid (minutes) and produces immediate symptoms. In the upper airways this is associated with nasal itch, sneeze, and rhinorrhoea (which are all neurally mediated), as well as with nasal obstruction (which is vascular in origin). In the lower airways mediator release is associated with bronchoconstriction and hypersecretion of mucus, giving rise to tightness in the chest, breathlessness, cough, and wheeze. The stimulation of sensory nerves with neuropeptide release (substance P and calcitonin gene related peptide) may enhance the response. During persistent exposure to an allergen, as occurs in seasonal and perennial allergic rhinitis and allergic asthma, there is also tissue accumulation of eosinophils. Activation of eosinophils with leukotriene release contributes to signs and symptoms of clinical disease, as does mediator release from activated epithelial cells.

Inflammatory cell accumulation and activation

Biopsy studies in asthma, rhinitis, and conjunctivitis specifically show an accumulation of effector cells in the epithelium, with an increase of mast cells, eosinophils, and basophils. The accumulation of inflammatory cells in the epithelium in patients with hay fever during the grass pollen season underlies the clinical observation of "priming," a situation in which patients' symptoms are more severe later in the season than at the start, despite the same pollen concentration. Eosinophil accumulation, along with an increase in T lymphocytes, is evident in the dermis in atopic dermatitis (eczema).

The local release of cytokines and chemokines (chemotactic cytokines) from activated T lymphocytes, mast cells, and epithelial cells can account for this accumulation of inflammatory cells in the airways. For T cell activation there has to be a specific interaction between the T cell and an antigen presenting cell, which processes the allergen and presents it to the T cell in a modified format. The major antigen presenting cells in the airways and skin are dendritic or Langerhans' cells, and these are found to accumulate in the

---

Airways inflammation underlies clinical disease expression in allergic asthma and rhinitis

---

Contribution of mediators to signs and symptoms of disease

Mediator	Signs and symptoms	
	Rhinitis	Asthma
Histamine	Itch; sneeze; rhinorrhoea; obstruction	Bronchoconstriction; plasma protein exudation; mucus secretion
Leukotrienes	Possible rhinorrhoea; obstruction	Bronchoconstriction; plasma protein exudation; mucus secretion
Kinins	Obstruction	Bronchoconstriction; cough
Prostaglandins	Obstruction	Bronchoconstriction (prostaglandin $F_2\alpha$, prostaglandin D_2); anti-bronchoconstrictor (prostaglandin E_2); cough (prostaglandin $F_2\alpha$)
Endothelin	Itch; sneeze; rhinorrhoea	Bronchoconstriction

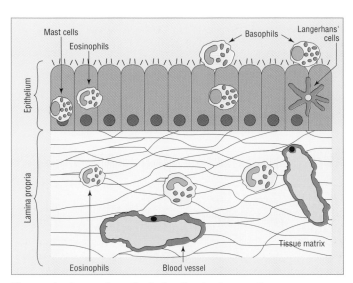

Changes in the number of cells in allergic airways disease: an accumulation in the epithelium of the major effector cells of the allergic reaction (mast cells, eosinophils, and basophils) and antigen presenting cells (Langerhans' cells); and an increase in eosinophils in the submucosa and in a subpopulation of fibroblasts ("myofibroblasts") in the tissue matrix (not illustrated)

airway epithelium and have been reported to express high affinity IgE receptors. There is evidence in perennial asthma, perennial rhinitis, and acute atopic dermatitis for an increase in T cells exhibiting a Th2 cytokine profile.

Th2 cytokines act in concert to promote an accumulation of eosinophils in the airways through endothelial activation and the enhanced adherence of these leucocytes to the vascular endothelium. They do this by increasing the eosinophil chemotactic response to chemokines, stimulating marrow generation of progenitor cells, and decreasing tissue removal by inhibiting apoptosis (cell death). The directed movement of these cells, and of mast cells, basophils, T lymphocytes, and Langerhans' cells, is regulated by chemokine release from activated epithelial cells. Epithelial cells represent the primary mucosal interface with the environment, and the activation of epithelial cells by other environmental factors, such as pollutants or viral infection, provides a basis for their interaction in allergic airways disease. This epithelial activation in allergic airways disease is indirectly reflected by raised concentrations of nitric oxide in exhaled air, as the inducible form of an enzyme, nitric oxide synthase, is up regulated and may provide a potentially measurable marker to monitor the impact of anti-inflammatory treatment.

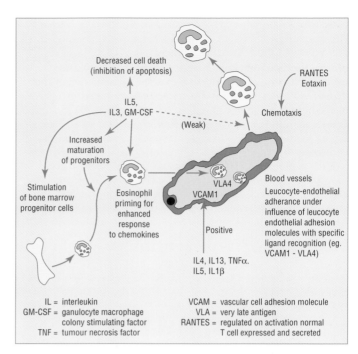

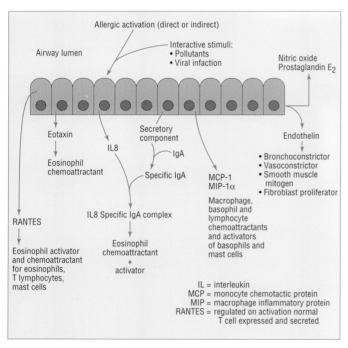

Epithelial activation and airway inflammation: products generated by epithelial cells in allergic airways disease and their relation to inflammatory cell recruitment

Processes involved in recruitment and retention of eosinophils in the airways. Cytokines (predominantly interleukin 5) stimulate bone marrow progenitor cells, cell priming, and adherence of leucocytes to the endothelium. Cytokines stimulate the endothelial cells, with specific leucocyte endothelial cell adhesion molecule expression and binding to cell-surface expressed ligands. Chemokines influence cell chemotaxis

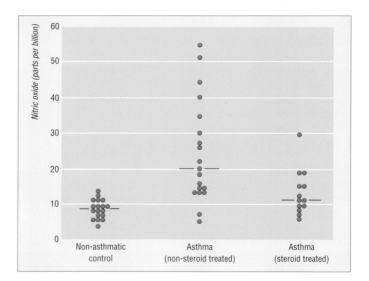

Measurement of nitric oxide in oral exhaled air in mixed expired air sample in non-asthmatic healthy controls (n = 18), asthmatic patients not treated with steroids (n = 19), and asthmatic patients receiving inhaled steroid treatment (n = 13). Horizontal lines indicate median values for each group

Implications for treatment

Allergen avoidance

The first step in management once allergy has been diagnosed is allergen avoidance. Allergen avoidance can help to reduce disease severity and minimise treatment in patients with asthma, rhinitis, and atopic dermatitis. The essential principle is thus to identify the provoking allergens and where possible ensure that the patient avoids them. Identification is based on clinical history and on objective assessment of the presence of

> **Allergen avoidance can be life saving in patients with anaphylaxis**

specific IgE. Avoidance protocols will be discussed in a later article.

Pharmacotherapy

Adrenaline is first line treatment for anaphylaxis and is most effective when administered early. Glucocorticoids represent the most efficacious treatment when administered as regular prophylactics. They regulate gene transcription and down regulate cytokine and chemokine synthesis, thus indirectly inhibiting cell recruitment and cell activation. Glucocorticoid treatment reduces epithelial and endothelial cell activation; reduces accumulation of epithelial mast cells, eosinophils, and Langerhans' cells; enhances eosinophil apoptosis; and reduces T cell and mast cell cytokine generation. The treatment is best administered topically to the airways and skin to reduce the possibility of systemic side effects.

Cromones are less effective as anti-inflammatory agents as they have a more restricted profile of effects. Specific end organ receptor antagonists (H₁ antihistamines, anticholinergic agents, and leukotriene receptor antagonists) and functional antagonists (β adrenoceptor agonists (bronchodilators) and α agonists (vasoconstrictor decongestants)) will be limited by their specificity of action, although the oral treatments have value in targeting upper and lower airways as well as the conjunctiva.

Histamine is a dominant mediator in the upper airways (H₁ receptor mediated), and leukotrienes are a significant contributor to lower airways disease (leukotriene C₄ and D₄ receptor mediated).

The importance in asthma of targeting the airway inflammation rather than the end organ effects is emphasised by the British guidelines on asthma management as this approach not only leads to improved disease control but also can prevent irreversible loss of lung function if used early in disease management. This loss of lung function is attributable to chronic structural airway changes that develop if allergic inflammation is left untreated.

Immunotherapy

Allergen immunotherapy is the repeated administration of low doses of an allergen to which an individual is sensitised in a stepwise incremental pattern, usually by subcutaneous injection, over some years (usually three to five). This is done to influence the state of immunological and clinical tolerance. This treatment is thought to act via either immune deviation of T lymphocyte responses from a Th2 to a Th1 profile or by the induction of T cell unresponsiveness (anergy). Although immunotherapy is well established for seasonal allergic rhinitis, it is a less well proved approach for house dust mite sensitive asthma and rhinitis. It is the primary treatment to consider for modifying sensitisation to bee and wasp venom.

Future approaches

Treatments are being developed that focus on inhibiting the interaction between IgE and allergen; inhibiting cytokine or chemokine function (such as a monoclonal antibody to interleukin 5 or a chemokine receptor antagonist); inhibiting T cell activation; modifying endothelial leucocyte interactions (very late antigen 4 antagonist); and modifying epithelial cell activation. The long term future must, however, depend on a better understanding of the basis for the increase in allergic diseases so that they can be prevented, rather than depending on secondary disease control.

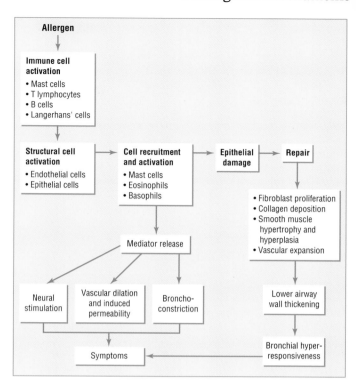

Progression of the allergic process in the airways and the relation of this process to inflammatory cell recruitment and symptom expression

Further reading

- Colloff MJ, Ayres J, Carswell F, Howarth PH, Merrett TG, Mitchell EB, et al. The control of allergens of dust mites and domestic pets: a position paper. *Clin Exp Allergy* 1992;22(suppl 2):1-28
- Jarvis D, Burney P. Epidemiology of atopy and atopic disease. In: Kay AB, ed. *Allergy and allergic disease*. Oxford: Blackwell Scientific, 1997:1208-26
- Howarth PH. Cellular basis for allergic rhinitis. *Allergy* 1995;50(suppl 23):6-10
- Barnes PJ. NFkB—a pivotal transcription factor in chronic inflammatory diseases. *N Engl J Med* 1997;336:1066-71
- British guidelines on asthma management. 1995 review and position statement. *Thorax* 1997;52(suppl 1):S1-21

Mikola Jacobson and Stephen Durham provided the histology photographs.

5 Summer hay fever

Stephen Durham

Summer hay fever causes considerable morbidity and affects quality of life at a time usually considered as the best of the year. Its prevalence has increased over the past 20 years despite falling pollen counts.

> **Antihistaminesd and nasal corticosteroid sprays are forst line treatment**

Environmental triggers

The main cause of hay fever in Britain is grass pollen, particularly perennial rye *(Lolium perenne)* and timothy grass *(Phleum pratense)*. Symptoms peak during June and July. Symptoms in spring are commonly due to tree pollens, whereas symptoms in late summer and autumn may be due to weed pollens and mould spores. Rape seed may also provoke symptoms of rhinitis, although usually through irritant rather than allergic mechanisms. It has been suggested that emissions of nitrogen dioxide and ozone from vehicle exhausts have been increasing the sensitivity to airborne allergens.

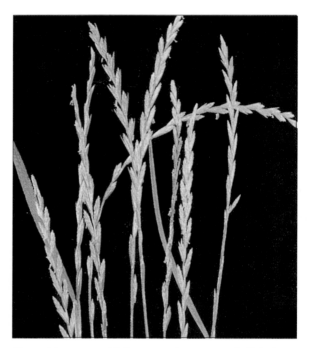

Perennial rye grass (*Lolium perenne*)—common in Britain

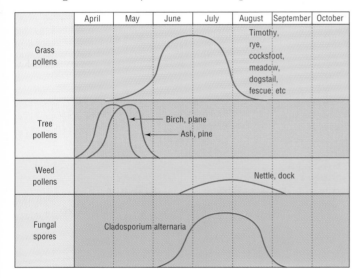

Pollen calendar for Britain

Mechanisms of rhinitis

The symptoms of rhinitis are caused by an interaction between grass pollen and IgE on the surface of sensitised mucosal mast cells (type 1 hypersensitivity). The cells release mediators such as histamine and leukotrienes, which produce itch, sneeze, watery anterior nasal discharge, nasal congestion, and symptoms affecting the eyes.

Allergens are also recognised and processed by mucosal dendritic cells (Langerhans' cells) or macrophages, which then stimulate T lymphocytes to release interleukins, which promote tissue eosinophilia and IgE production. These compounds act to produce ongoing rhinitis, symptoms of blockage, impaired sense of smell, and nasal hyperreactivity (an exaggerated nasal response to environmental irritants such as cold air, perfume, or tobacco smoke).

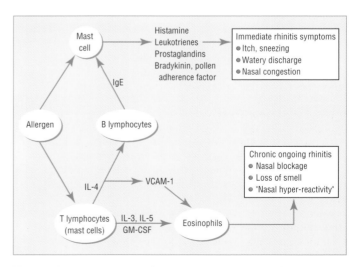

Hypothesis on mechanisms of summer hay fever (rationale basis for treatment). IL = interleukin, VCAM = vascular cell adhesion molecules, GM-CSF = granulocyte macrophage colony stimulating factor

Diagnosis

Most patients present with the diagnostic symptoms of seasonal itching, sneezing, watery nasal discharge, and associated eye problems. The nose may be examined with an auriscope to exclude a structural problem. Skin prick tests are not usually needed for diagnosis, but a positive result may help to reinforce advice to take topical prophylaxis.

Drug treatment

Antihistamines

Oral antihistamines are effective in patients with mild to moderate disease, particularly in those whose main symptoms are palatal itch, sneezing, rhinorrhoea, or eye symptoms. Also some patients may prefer a tablet to topical applications. Antihistamines have little effect, however, on nasal blockage.

Terfenadine and astemizole are effective, and rarely cause drowsiness or anticholinergic side effects. With these drugs it is important to emphasise the manufacturers' instructions in view of the extremely rare complication of cardiac arrhythmias in overdose and, in the case of terfenadine, interactions with erythromycin or ketoconazole and grapefruit juice (which should not be given concurrently).

Newer alternatives including cetirizine, fexofenadine, and loratidine are at least as effective and do not have these interactions. Acrivastine is short acting and may be useful when symptoms are mild and episodic. The place of topical nasal antihistamines in hay fever is currently being evaluated.

Corticosteroids

Topical corticosteroids are extremely potent, with a low potential for systemic side effects. They are the best treatment for patients with moderate to severe nasal symptoms. Aqueous corticosteroids are better tolerated than those in fluorocarbon propellants and have a better local distribution in the nose. The side effects are minor—local irritation and occasional (in 5% of cases) bleeding. Treatment should be started before the beginning of the hay fever season for maximal effect. Patients should be given instruction on the importance of regular treatment and how to use the nasal spray.

Topical corticosteroids are effective against all nasal symptoms, including nasal blockage. Although systemic absorption is negligible in adults, care should be taken when nasal steroids are given to children who are also taking inhaled steroids for asthma or topical steroids for eczema. Sodium cromoglycate two to four times daily is an alternative, particularly in children. Eye drops containing sodium cromoglycate, are effective in most patients (often within minutes) for allergic eye symptoms Nedocromil eye drops are longer acting and effective when taken twice daily.

Second line treatment

In patients who fail to respond to antihistamines or topical corticosteroids, a short course of an oral corticosteroid (say, prednisolone 20mg for five days) may produce rapid relief of symptoms. This is particularly effective when the nose is completely obstructed as topical treatment will not gain access to the nose.

An alternative is to use a topical decongestant short term to allow penetration of topical corticosteroids. Ipratropium bromide may have a role when watery rhinorrhoea is pronounced.

In general it is important to establish which are the patient's dominant symptoms and, particularly for severe symptoms, to match the treatment to the symptoms.

Diagnosis of hay fever

History	Prominent itch or sneezing and associated eye symptoms
Nasal examination	Pale, bluish, swollen mucosa (only if symptomatic at time)
Skin prick test or radioallergosorbent test	Not essential, although of educational value and reinforces oral advice

---

> **Diagnosis of summer hay fever is usually straightforward**

Stepwise approach to treatment of summer hay fever

Allergen avoidance (if appropriate)

Mild disease or with occasional symptoms
- Rapid onset, oral, non-sedating histamine H_1 antagonists when the patient is symptomatic; or
- Antihistamine or cromoglycate topically to eyes or nose, or both

Moderate disease with prominent nasal symptoms
- Topical nasal steroid daily (start early in the season); plus
- Antihistamine or cromoglycate topically to eyes

Moderate disease with prominent eye symptoms
- Oral, non-sedating histamine H_1 antagonists daily; or
- Topical nasal steroid and sodium cromoglycate topically to eyes

If above are ineffective, check compliance and consider:
- Nasal examination
- Allergy tests
- Additional pharmacotherapy—for example, short course of oral steroids
- Immunotherapy (requires referral to specialist)

Effects of drugs on nasal symptoms in adults

	Itch or sneezing	Discharge	Blockage	Impaired smell
Topical corticosteroids	+ + +	+ + +	+ +	+
Oral antihistamines	+ + +	+ +	+/−	−
Sodium cromoglycate*	+	+	+/−	−
Ipratropium bromide	−	+ + +	−	−
Topical decongestants	−	−	+ + +	−
Oral corticosteroids	+ + +	+ + +	+ + +	+ +

*First line treatment in children.

17

Avoiding allergens

Patients with allergies are usually advised to avoid the provoking allergen. It is, however, controversial whether this should be routinely recommended for pollen allergy. As hay fever is usually not severe or life threatening, drugs can allow patients to lead a normal life without unnecessary restrictions. But patients with debilitating symptoms may benefit from simple advice. Pollen counts at ground level are highest during the evening and at night, when open grassy spaces should be avoided.

Immunotherapy

Most patients with hay fever will have their symptoms controlled by the above measures. Patients whose symptoms remain uncontrolled may benefit from "allergen injection immunotherapy." This form of treatment is performed only in specialised centres. Careful selection of patients for this treatment is essential, and immunotherapy is contraindicated in those with chronic asthma. Indications and guidelines for immunotherapy in Britain were the subject of a recent report by the British Society for Allergy and Clinical Immunology.

The pollen calendar is adapted with permission from Varney (*Clin Exp Allergy* 1991;21:757). The diagram showing the mechanisms of summer hay fever and the box on the stepwise approach to the treatment are adapted with permission from Lund et al (*Allergy* 1994;49(suppl 19):1-34).

How to avoid pollen
- Keep windows in cars and buildings shut
- Wear glasses or sunglasses
- Avoid open grassy places, particularly in the evening and at night
- Use a car with a pollen filter
- Check for pollen counts in the media
- During the peak season take a holiday by the sea or abroad

Grass pollen immunotherapy
- Immunotherapy should be considered in patients with summer hay fever uncontrolled by antiallergy drugs
- It should be administered only in hospital or specialised clinics with immediate access to resuscitative facilities
- Patients should be kept under observation for the first 60 minutes after injections
- Patients with asthma should not be given grass pollen immunotherapy
- Allergen extracts used should be biologically standardised

Further reading
- Howarth PH. Allergic rhinitis: a rational choice of treatment. *Respir Med* 1989;83:179-88
- Naclerio RM. Allergic rhinitis. *N Engl J Med* 1991;325:860
- Lund V on behalf of the International Rhinitis Management Working Group. International consensus report on the diagnosis and management of rhinitis. *Allergy* 1994;49(suppl 19):1-34
- Frew AJ on behalf of a British Society for Allergy and Clinical Immunology Working Party. Injection immunotherapy. *BMJ* 1993;307:919-22

6 Perennial rhinitis

I S Mackay, S R Durham

Perennial rhinitis may be defined clinically as an inflammatory condition of the nose characterised by nasal obstruction, sneezing, itching, or rhinorrhoea, occurring for an hour or more on most days throughout the year. In one study in London of adults between the ages of 16 and 65 years, the prevalence of rhinitis was 16%; of these, 8% had perennial symptoms, 6% perennial and seasonal symptoms, and 2% seasonal symptoms alone. As with asthma, both seasonal and perennial rhinitis seem to be increasing.

Classification

Allergic rhinitis—Perennial allergic rhinitis can be more difficult to diagnose than seasonal allergy, particularly if the patient presents with secondary symptoms of sinusitis and a "permanent cold." The most common allergen to account for perennial allergic symptoms is the house dust mite (*Dermatophagoides pteronyssinus*). Other frequent causes are animals: particularly cats, dogs, and horses.

Occupational rhinitis may result from allergy to airborne agents in the workplace—for example, laboratory animals and latex.

Infective rhinitis—Infective rhinitis may be acute or chronic. Chronic symptoms may be due to specific infections, such as fungi or tuberculosis. Chronic infection may also be the result of a host defence deficiency; this may be systemic (for example, panhypogammaglobulinaemia, IgA deficiency, or AIDS) or a local problem (for example, primary ciliary dyskinesia).

Other factors—Other non-allergic, non-infective factors may be involved (see box).

Differential diagnosis

Structural abnormalities of the nose include deviation of the nose or septum, enlarged middle and inferior turbinates, adenoidal hypertrophy (particularly in children; rare in adults), and choanal atresia. The ostiomeatal complex is the area lying between the middle and inferior turbinates and the natural ostium of the maxillary sinus. It is this area which drains and aerates the maxillary sinus, the anterior ethmoidal sinuses, and the frontal sinus. Obstruction in this area, whether structural or secondary to an inflammatory condition, will predispose to sinusitis.

Nasal polyps result from inflammation of the mucosal lining of the sinuses; the lining prolapses down, particularly from the anterior ethmoidal sinuses through the middle meatus to obstruct the nasal airway. Allergy does not seem to be an important factor. Nasal polyps in children are rare and are almost invariably associated with cystic fibrosis. A strong association exists between nasal polyps, asthma, and sensitivity to aspirin (Samter's triad).

Granulomatous rhinitis may be associated with Wegener's granulomatosis and sarcoidosis.

Primary atopic rhinitis is characterised by nasal congestion, hyposmia, and an unpleasant smell (ozoena), resulting from a progressive atrophy of the nasal mucosa and underlying bone. Secondary atrophic rhinitis may result from radical surgery, infections, irradiation, and trauma.

Non-allergic, non-infective rhinitis★

- *Idiopathic rhinitis* refers to a heterogeneous group of patients with nasal hyperresponsiveness to non-specific triggers such as strong smells (eg, perfumes, bleach, and solvents), tobacco smoke, vehicle exhaust fumes, and changes in environmental temperature and humidity in the absence of an identifiable underlying cause
- *Non-allergic rhinitis with eosinophilia syndrome* (NARES) is characterised by nasal eosinophilia (usually in young women) with perennial nasal symptoms with negative results on skin prick testing and normal IgE concentrations. Patients usually respond well to topical corticosteroids
- *Hormonal rhinitis* can occur during pregnancy, puberty, hypothyroidism, and acromegaly. Postmenopausal women may develop atrophic changes, elderly men sometimes watery rhinorrhoea ("old man's drip")
- *Drug induced rhinitis* is associated with several drugs. β sympathomimetic receptor antagonists (β blockers) and angiotensin converting enzyme inhibitors have been associated with nasal symptoms, as have topical ophthalmic β blockers, chlorpromazine, oral contraceptives, aspirin, and other non-steroidal anti-inflammatory agents
- *Food induced rhinitis* Gustatory rhinorrhoea may occur during consumption of hot and spicy foods. Non-IgE mediated hypersensitivity may result from food colourings and preservatives. Alcohol, in addition to the mechanisms above, also acts as a vasodilator, which may result in nasal obstruction
- *Emotional factors* including stress and sexual arousal can affect the nose, probably due to autonomic stimulation

★Poorly understood and more difficult to identify specific causes

---

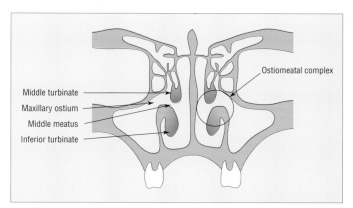

Nasal cavity showing ostimeatal complex. It is the final common pathway draining the maxillary sinus, the anterior ethmoidal sinus, and the frontal sinus

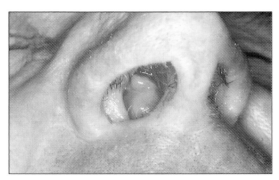

Nasal polyp

Leaking of cerebrospinal fluid will present with watery rhinorrhoea, often unilateral. It is usually associated with trauma (including surgical trauma) or neoplasia, but spontaneous leaking may occur.

> **Nasal neoplasms are rare; consider patients with unilateral symptoms of nasal obstruction, pain, or bleeding**

History and examination

Taking a history need not be time consuming. A glance at the classification and differential diagnosis will suggest the most important questions.

Rare, sinister causes for rhinitis need to be excluded. Unilateral symptoms should always be regarded with suspicion, particularly if associated with symptoms of increasing nasal obstruction, blood stained nasal discharge, or facial pain.

Ear, nose, and throat surgeons examine the nose with a head mirror or headlight and a nasal speculum, but increasingly this is supplemented by rigid or flexible nasendoscopy. In general practice, the nose can be examined with an auriscope fitted with the largest speculum. It is easy to confuse a large, swollen, oedematous inferior or middle turbinate with a polyp; polyps, however, unlike turbinates, are usually pale grey, translucent, and mobile and lack any sensation on gentle probing.

Investigation

Perennial allergic and non-allergic rhinitis may require no specific investigations other than skin prick testing, which has been fully discussed in an earlier article in this series. If the history or examination suggests that other factors need to be excluded, the patient may require a variety of investigations, depending on the history and clinical findings.

Special tests
In addition to routine full blood count and eosinophil count, immunoglobulin concentrations should be checked. Blood tests for antineutrophil cytoplasmic antibody and angiotensin converting enzyme may be indicated if, respectively, Wegener's granuloma or nasal sarcoidosis is suspected. It is also important to consider whether the patient may have AIDS or be compromised by treatment with immunosupressant drugs. When skin prick tests are not available or not possible for other reasons, blood allergen specific IgE concentrations may be determined (with the radioallergosorbent test).

Imaging
Plain *x* ray films of the sinuses can be misleading. Computed tomography of the sinuses in the coronal plane has become the standard international imaging method.

Nasal mucociliary clearance
Nasal mucociliary clearance is assessed simply, by measuring the time taken for the patient to detect a sweet taste after a 0.5 mm particle of saccharin is placed on the mucosa of the inferior turbinate. If the test result is abnormal, further assessment of ciliary function involves taking a brushing of the nasal mucosa overlying the inferior turbinate and measuring the frequency of the beating cilia detected with a microscope attached to a photometric cell (normal range 12-15 Hz).

Nasal airway assessment
Peak nasal inspiratory flow can be measured with a modified peak flow meter. This test is easy and inexpensive to perform, but forced inspiration may be associated with significant vestibular collapse. Despite this, the results compare favourably with rhinomanometry.

Taking a history
- Patient's account of symptoms
- How long has the condition been present?
- Impact on lifestyle: how frequent and severe is it? Does it affect work, school, leisure time, sleep?
- Seasonal or perennial?
- Trigger factors: allergic or non-allergic?
- Exposure to allergens through occupation or hobbies?
- Allergens in the home
- Does patient have history of asthma, eczema, rhinitis?
- Drug or food induced?
- Family history
- Treatment: compliance, efficacy, side effects
- What is the main symptom?

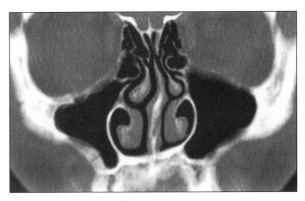

Computed tonogram of normal paranasal sinuses

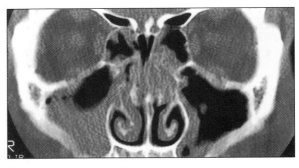

Computed tomogram of paranasal sinuses with increased opacity of maxillary and ethmoidal sinuses and obstruction of ostiomeatal complex

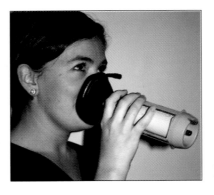

Modified peak flow meter for measuring peak nasal inspiratory flow

Rhinomanometry records resistance in the nasal airway by measuring nasal airflow with a face mask, pneumotachograph, and pressure gradient from the front to the back of the nose via a manometer.

Acoustic rhinometry measures neither flow nor pressure, but cross sectional areas of the nasal airway. A sound pulse is passed into the nose, the reflected signal of which is recorded by a microphone and analysed in such a way that it is possible to determine the area in the nasal cavity as a function of distance.

Olfactory tests

Olfactory thresholds can be assessed by testing the patient with serial dilutions of odours such as PM-carbinol (phenylethyl methyl ethyl carbinol) (Olfacto-Labs, USA). Alternatively, "scratch and sniff" tests use cards impregnated with microencapsulated odorants. The Pocket Smell Test (Sensonics, USA), for example, presents three different odours that can be released by scratching with the tip of a pencil and choosing from a list of four possible answers. One or more incorrect reponses suggests olfactory dysfunction, and the 40 item Smell Identification Test (Sensonics) should then be administered.

Swabs, smears, and biopsies

With infective symptoms, swabs for culture and sensitivity may be useful, though a swab taken from the nose will not necessarily correlate with samples taken directly from the sinuses. Nasal smears for cytology may show high concentrations of eosinophils, and biopsies for histology may be indicated when investigating granulomatous conditions—for example, Wegener's granulomatosis and sarcoidosis—or excluding neoplastic disease.

Treatment

Allergen avoidance

Perennial allergic rhinitis due to house dust mite allergy may be effectively controlled by avoidance measures. Patients who are found to be allergic to animals should, if possible, avoid them completely.

Medical treatment

Antihistamines

Antihistamines are highly effective in controlling itching, sneezing, and watery rhinorrhoea but less effective for nasal obstruction. However, they do have the advantage of controlling eye symptoms as well as nasal symptoms. The modern generation of non-sedating antihistamines are both effective and safe, although terfenadine should not be taken in conjunction with macrolide antibiotics (for example, erythromycin and clarithromycin) or antifungal agents (ketaconazole and related drugs) as serious cardiac toxicity has very rarely been reported. Topical antihistamines (for example, azelastine and levocobastine) are also effective.

Topical steroids

Topical steroids are highly effective for all symptoms of allergic and non-allergic perennial rhinitis and will usually control nasal obstruction, itching, sneezing, and watery rhinorrhoea. The modern topical steroids are safe for long term use and have no significant side effects. Treatment can be continued for several years if necessary, and alternative medical or surgical treatment need be considered only if symptoms fail to respond. Occasionally, topical steroids may be associated with dryness, crusting, and bleeding from the nose, in which case treatment should be discontinued for a few days and then restarted.

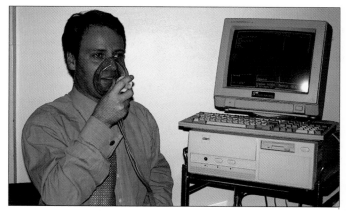

Rhinomanometry: flow is recorded via a face mask and pneumotachograph, and pressure change is measured with a manometer via a tube either to one nostril (unilateral) or through the mouth to the back of the nose (bilateral)

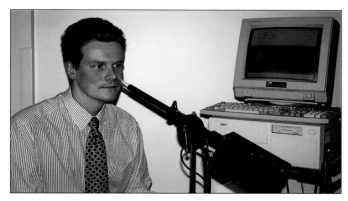

Acoustic rhinometry measures cross sectional areas of the nasal airway

Desensitisation

- Desensitisation for pollen allergy for and bee and wasp venom anaphylaxis is highly effective
- Perennial rhinitis is often multifactorial such that desensitisation is less effective and seldom used in Britain

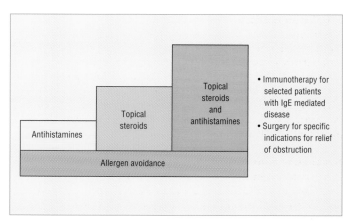

Stepwise approach to treatment of perennial rhinitis

Sodium cromoglycate

Sodium cromoglycate is more effective in atopic than non-atopic patients. It has no known side effects but is less effective than antihistamines and corticosteroids and does require frequent use (up to five times daily), which may compromise compliance. Topical sodium cromoglycate eye drops are highly effective for allergic conjunctivitis. Topical nedocromil eye drops are also effective and have a longer duration of effect (up to 12 hours).

Topical anticholinergics

Ipratropium bromide is effective in controlling watery rhinorrhoea, particularly if this is the only symptom. The dose may need to be titrated against symptoms.

Nasal decongestants

Topical nasal decongestants may be useful at the start of treatment to "open up" the nose and improve penetration of topical corticosteroids, when flying, or for upper respiratory tract infections. They should only be used for short courses (preferably no more than 2 weeks), however, to avoid the risk of developing "rhinitis medicamentosa" (rebound congestion).

Surgical treatment

- The first line of treatment for allergic or non-allergic perennial rhinitis is usually medical
- When drugs fail, surgery may be indicated
- Surgical reduction of the inferior turbinates or correction of a deviated nasal septum or nose may be required to improve the airway or at least to improve access for topical medical treatment
- Surgery continues to have a major role in the management of nasal polyps and sinusitis when these conditions fail to respond to medical treatment
- The management of nasal polyps and sinusitis has improved with the introduction of minimally invasive endoscopic sinus surgery

Further reading

- Lund V, Aaronson D, Bousquet J, Dahl R, Davies RJ, Durham SR, et al. International consensus report on the diagnosis and management of rhinitis. *Allergy* 1994;49(suppl 19)
- Sibbald B, Rink E. Epidemiology of seasonal and perennial rhinitis. Clinical presentation and medical history. *Thorax* 1991;46:859-901
- Fleming DM, Crombie DL. Prevalence of asthma and hayfever in England and Wales. *BMJ* 1987;294:279-83
- Durham SR, Mackay IS. The nose. In: Brewis RAL, Corrin B, Geddes DM, eds. *Respiratory medicine*. 2nd ed. Vol 2. London: Saunders, 1995:1006-14

7 Allergic eye disease

Roger Buckley

Allergic eye disease ranges in effect from the inconvenient to the sight threatening. The common diseases are mild, do not affect the cornea, and can be manged without steroids. The rarer manifestations are severe, involve the cornea, and usually require the topical use of steroids.

Examination of the ocular surfaces

To examine the tarsal conjunctiva, which is the main site of allergic processes affecting the surface of the eye, it is necessary to evert the upper eyelid. This is easily done using a long thin object (e.g. a cotton bud) as a fulcrum at the top of the tarsal plate, while the eyelashes are pulled forward and up. This will not hurt if the patient looks steadily down. The conjunctiva is best examined at the slit lamp, but a naked-eye examination can provide useful information.

Seasonal allergic conjunctivitis

Up to 21% of adults in this country report symptoms attributable to seasonal allergic conjunctivitis. In some this is merely the ocular component of hay fever, while in others only the eyes are affected. The mucosal mechanisms are probably similar to those proposed for allergic rhinitis (see chapter 5 on Summer hay fever) and the environmental triggers are the same: tree pollens in April and May, grass pollens in June and July, and weed pollens and fungal spores in July and August. Release of histamine and leukotrienes into the tear film produces the characteristic symptoms of itching, watering, and redness. The clinical signs are few, being restricted to hyperaemia and oedema of the tarsal conjunctival surfaces. It is not yet clear whether, or to what extent, this disease is controlled by T-lymphocytes.

Diagnosis

This is made on the basis of a typical history. Skin prick tests and conjunctival challenge tests are rarely necessary

Management

Seasonal allergic conjunctivitis can be managed either topically, with eye drops, or systemically. Topical treatment using the mast cell stabilisers sodium cromoglycate (e.g. Opticrom), nedocromil sodium (Rapitil), or lodoxamide (Alomide) is rapidly effective and safe. Nedocromil can be used twice daily, while the others must generally be used four times daily. Topical antihistamines, such as levocabastine, an H_1-receptor antagonist, can also be used. Topical steroid preparations are very effective, but the risk of unwanted, sight-threatening effects (glaucoma, cataract, enhancement of infection) is high and therefore unacceptable. Many patients are happy with the effect provided by oral antihistamines such as terfenadine, astemizole, and cetirizine, and such treatment is particularly appropriate when there are nasal symptoms also.

Allergic eye diseases: population affected, incidence, morbidity, steroid need

Disease	Those affected	UK Incidence in	Morbidity	Need of steroid
• SAC	• Young adults	• Common	• Low	• Zero
• PAC	• Similar to SAC	• Uncommon	• Medium	• Zero/low
• VKC	• Children	• Rare	• High	• High
• AKC	• Adults	• Rare	• High	• High
• GPC	• CL wearers	• Fairly common	• Medium	• Zero/low

AKC, atopic keratoconjunctivitis; GPC, giant papillary conjunctivitis; PAC, perennial allergic conjunctivitis; SAC, seasonal allergic conjunctivitis; VKC, vernal keratoconjunctivitis; CL, contact lens

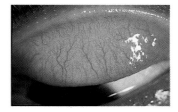

The everted upper tarsus in Seasonal Allergic conjunctivitis. The appearance is virtually normal

---

Drug Treatment of Seasonal Allergic Conjunctivitis

- topical mast cell stabilisers
- topical antihistamines
- antihistamine tablets

Perennial allergic conjunctivitis

This condition, the ocular equivalent of perennial allergic rhinitis, is much rarer than the seasonal disease. The symptoms and signs are similar but milder, and show seasonal variation. In this country, the main responsible allergen is the house dust mite. A high level of HDM-specific IgE (which is locally secreted) is found in the tears. Allergen avoidance measures are appropriate here (mite-proof mattress covers, 'clean' vacuum cleaners, etc.); otherwise, the treatment is as for seasonal allergic conjunctivitis.

> **Allergen avoidance measures and drug therapy are complementary in the management of Perennial allergic conjunctivitis**

Vernal keratoconjunctivitis

This is a rare but serious disease affecting some atopic children. Boys are much more often affected than girls. In most, the condition begins before the age of 10 years, and usually remits around puberty. It may sometimes metamorphose into atopic keratoconjunctivitis.

Diagnosis
The symptoms, which usually occur in spring or early summer (though in severe cases they continue year-round), are itching, watering, stickiness, and difficulty with opening the eyes on awaking. When the cornea is involved, blurred vision, pain and photophobia result. The signs consist of 'giant' (i.e. greater than 1 mm in diameter) papillary hyperplasia of the upper tarsal conjunctival surfaces, inflammation at the limbus (corneo–scleral junction), and erosion of the corneal epithelium. A stringy mucous exudate is often present on the eye and under the lids. Corneal involvement, if severe or prolonged, can cause scarring and loss of visual acuity. Scarring results in the conjunctiva also, but this does not produce the cicatrisation or the reduced tear production that are commonly associated with chronic conjunctival inflammation.

Management
Topical steroid preparations are usually needed, so regular screening for adverse effects is mandatory; vernal keratoconjunctivitis should therefore be managed by the ophthalmologist. Opticrom and other mast cell stabilisers are usually prescribed also, as they reduce the steroid requirement and, in some mild cases, may be sufficient on their own. More recently, cyclosporin eye drops have been shown to be effective, as might have been anticipated in a disease which is driven by T-lymphocyte activity. No commercial preparation is yet available and the experimental formulations (in oil, as the drug is insoluble in water) tend to be irritant. Mucolytic drops (acetyl cysteine 5% or 10%) are often helpful in controlling the symptoms attributable to the abnormal mucus.

Atopic keratoconjunctivitis

This rare condition is potentially the most severe manifestation of allergic disease in the eye. It is a lifelong condition affecting some atopic adults, and indeed may evolve from pre-existing vernal disease.

Diagnosis
The symptoms are perpetual ocular itching, soreness, a feeling of dryness, and impaired vision. The signs include eczema of the eyelids, chronic lid margin infection, chronic cicatrising conjunctivitis, tear abnormality, and progressive scarring and vascularisation of the cornea. There are associations with keratoconus and atopic cataract.

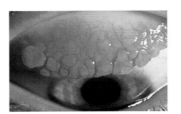

Giant papillary hyperplasia of the everted upper tarsus in Vernal keratoconjunctivitis. Here the condition is quiescent; the patient is symptom-free

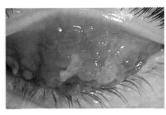

Active Vernal keratoconjunctivitis with severe conjunctival inflammation affecting the everted upper tarsus

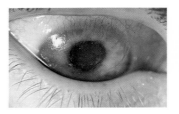

Corneal epithelial erosion in active Vernal keratoconjunctivitis

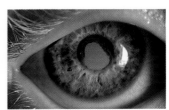

Corneal plaque in Vernal keratoconjunctivitis

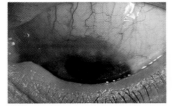

Severe limbal inflammation in Vernal keratoconjunctivitis

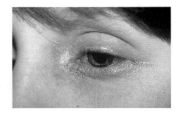

Lid eczema in Atopic keratoconjunctivitis

> **Corticosteroid eye drops should *only* be prescribed under regular supervision of an ophthalmologist**

Management

Like vernal disease, this condition should be managed by the ophthalmologist. Topical steroid will be required, though not constantly. Treatment of the infected lid margins, with topical or (more effectively) systemic antibiotic, may help considerably to reduce the symptoms. Opticrom and other mast cell stabilisers may help also. The beneficial effect of topical cyclosporin was recently shown in this condition also, though the irritancy of oily solutions to chronically inflamed ocular surfaces can be problematical.

Giant papillary conjunctivitis

First described in 1974 in soft contact lens wearers, this condition has since been identified wherever there is contact between a foreign surface and the ocular mucous membrane. Some of the most affected patients are those who must wear artificial eyes.

Diagnosis

Contact lens wearers complain of ocular itching or discomfort. Wearing times are reduced, and there is an excessive mucous discharge. Lenses may tend to displace from centration on the eye. The symptoms abate briefly if a new lens (or prosthesis) is substituted. The upper tarsal conjunctiva shows giant papillary hyperplasia which strongly resembles that seen in vernal keratoconjunctivitis. There is no corneal involvement, and limbal inflammation is rare.

Management

The fit, condition, and cleaning schedule of the contact lenses or prosthesis should be assessed. Sometimes it is appropriate to switch lens wearers to disposable lenses, perhaps even daily disposable lenses, if lens deposits are a problem. If medication is indicated, Opticrom or similar drugs may be given. Topical steroid is to be avoided, except in wearers of prostheses, where no eye exists to be damaged by unwanted effects.

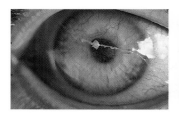

Adherent mucus and corneal vascularisation in Atopic keratoconjunctivitis

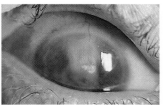

Corneal scarring in Atopic keratoconjunctivitis

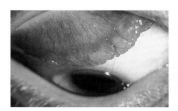

Giant Papillary Conjunctivitis of the upper border of the upper tarsus in a contact lens wearer

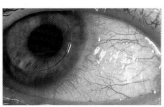

Limbal inflammation in a wearer of rigid corneal contact lenses

Further reading

Hingorani M, Lightman S. Therapeutic options in ocular allergic disease. *Drugs* 1995; **50**(2): 208–21.

Buckley R. Vernal keratoconjunctivitis. *Int Ophthalmol Clin* 1988; **28**(4): 303–8.

Buckley R. Diagnosis and treatment of atopic eye disease (Editorial). *Clin Exp Allergy* 1992; **22**: 887–8.

Galindez O. Kaufman H. Coping with the itchy-burnies: the management of allergic conjunctivitis (Guest Editorial). *Ophthalmology* 1996; **103**(9): 1335–6.

8 Asthma and allergy

A J Newman Taylor

Definitions and distinctions

Asthma

Asthma is commonly defined as a narrowing of the airways that is reversible over short periods of time, either spontaneously or as a result of treatment. This clinical definition (which characterises asthma as reversible airway narrowing) distinguishes it from other predominantly irreversible causes of airway narrowing, such as chronic obstructive bronchiolitis and emphysema. Another cardinal characteristic of asthma is airway hyper-responsiveness, an exaggerated narrowing of the airways provoked by a variety of non-specific stimuli, such as exercise and cold air. The two defining characteristics of asthma—reversible airway narrowing and airway hyper-responsiveness—are manifestations of a characteristic pattern of airway inflammation (a Th2 lymphocyte dependent desquamative eosinophilic bronchitis).

Atopy

Atopy is the propensity to produce IgE antibody to allergens (antigens that stimulate the production of IgE antibodies) that are commonly encountered in the general environment—for example, pollens, mites, and moulds. Atopy is usually identified by the provocation of one or more immediate "weal and flare" responses in the skin to extracts of common inhalant allergens. Specific IgE antibody to common inhalant allergens can be found in the serum samples of atopic individuals, who may also have a raised serum concentration of total IgE.

The development of atopy is influenced by both genetic and environmental factors:
● The genetic basis of atopy is debated. Twin studies have consistently shown that atopy occurs more frequently in identical than non-identical twins. The findings in different family studies, however, have not identified a consistent pattern of inheritance. Recent molecular studies have suggested an association between atopy and polymorphisms of the high affinity IgE receptor on chromosome 11q (FCΣR1-β) and linkage with the interleukin 4 gene cluster on chromosome 5. It seems likely that atopy will eventually be associated with polymorphisms of several different genes.
● The twofold to threefold increase in the prevalence of asthma during the past 30 years has been accompanied by an increase in the prevalence of hay fever and eczema and of skin prick test responses to common inhalant allergens. The difference in the prevalence of asthma in children between cities in former East Germany (Leipzig and Halle) and West Germany (Munich) after reunification was wholly accounted for by the 2.5-fold greater prevalence of atopy in Munich. Changes in prevalence of this magnitude, which have occurred over decades, are too rapid to reflect differences in the genetic pool and are probably due to changes in important environmental determinants of atopy, possibly a decrease in respiratory infection in early life.

Allergy

The concept of allergy was proposed by Clemens Freiherr von Pirquet in 1906 as a "specific acquired altered reactivity which follows initial exposure to foreign protein," a description that encompasses both immunity and allergy. Although allergy is

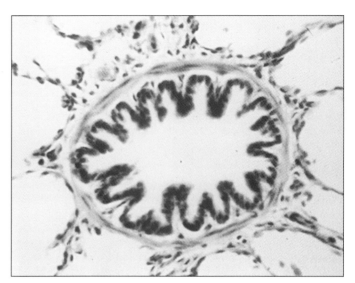

Normal bronchiole

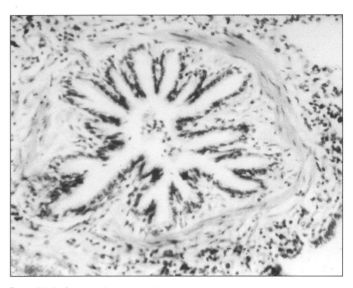

Bronchiole from asthmatic patient narrowed by eosinophilic infiltration, oedema, and increased smooth muscle

Allergy in atopic patients
● As well as asthma, eczema and hay fever are also manifestations of allergy in atopic patients
● Not all allergy is atopic—for example, drug reactions
● Not all allergic asthma is atopic—for example, asthma induced by the low molecular weight chemical sensitisers (such as isocyanates in two part polyurethane paints)
● Asthma can also be provoked through non-immunological reactions—for example, non-steroidal anti-inflammatory drugs and β blockers

now distinguished from immunity by a disproportionate injury to host tissue, the immunological reactions underlying both immune and allergic responses are the same; they differ only in their clinical outcome. This article is predominantly concerned with reactions associated with Th2 lymphocyte dependent IgE response whose outcome is characterised by local recruitment and activation of circulating blood eosinophils. This would be considered to be an immune response when directed against parasites such as shistosoma and filaria but an allergic response when directed against pollens and mites.

In this context, allergy is the clinical outcome of IgE associated reactions to common environmental allergens in atopic individuals. The characteristic allergic reactions in atopic individuals are eczema, hay fever, and asthma, which can, but do not by any means always, coexist in the same individual. Asthma may therefore be one of the manifestations of allergy in atopic individuals.

Asthma and allergy

Allergens and asthma
Asthma can be initiated and provoked by allergens in everyday life—outdoors, indoors, and at work. In patients whose asthma is provoked by protein allergens encountered in everyday life (such as pollens, mites, and moulds), extracts of relevant allergens in solution will elicit immediate skin test responses, and specific IgE antibody can be detected in their serum. This is also true for protein allergens that cause occupational asthma and for some low molecular weight chemicals encountered at work—for example, platinum salts, acid anhydrides, and reactive dyes (but not, for example, isocyanates, resin, wood dust). In general, evidence of specific IgE antibody, either from an immediate skin test response or specific IgE in serum, is a very sensitive test (that is, there are few false negatives) but also a non-specific test (that is, many false positives). A negative result is therefore more valuable than a positive result as it can exclude a specific cause of asthma, whereas a positive result is less reliable for identifying a specific cause and must always be interpreted in the context of the clinical history.

Allergens and asthma

Outdoors	Indoors
Pollens	*Mites*
Tree	Dermatophagoides pteronyssinus
Grass	and farinae (house dust mites)
Moulds	*Animals*
Alternaria alternata	Cats
Cladosporium herbatum	Dogs
Aspergillus fumigatus	Birds

Asthma and airway hyper-responsiveness
Exposure to allergens occurring naturally and in the laboratory can provoke airway narrowing and airway hyper-responsiveness. For example, patients allergic to ragweed pollen show a progressive increase in the severity of airway responsiveness during the ragweed season concurrently with the increase in the severity of their asthma.

Inhalation of soluble extracts of allergens provokes an immediate asthmatic response that peaks at about 20 minutes and resolves within about one hour. The provocation and severity of the immediate response is dependent on both the dose of inhaled allergen and the degree of airway hyper-responsiveness. In about 50% of patients a late asthmatic

Asthma in atopic patients
- Asthma is associated with atopy at all ages, although most strongly in children and young adults
- Atopic individuals may also have flexural eczema or hay fever concurrently, or have had them in the past
- The prevalence of asthma in different environments correlates with specific IgE antibody to the particular allergens present. For example, in cities in the United States asthma is associated in affluent areas with specific IgE to house dust mite and cat hair and in poor areas with specific IgE to house dust mite and cockroach
- Furthermore, the severity of asthma correlates with the concentration of specific allergens (such as house dust mite or cockroach) to which individuals are sensitised

---

Causes of occupational asthma

	Proteins	Low molecular weight chemicals
Animal	Excreta of rats, mice etc; locusts; grain mites	
Vegetable	Grain, flours; latex; green coffee bean; isphagula; latex	Plicatic acid (from western red cedar), pinewood resin
Microbial	Harvest moulds, Bacillus subtilis enzymes (in detergents)	Antibiotics—eg. penicillins, cephalosporins
Mineral		Acid anhydrides, isocyanates, complex platinium salts, polyamines, reactive dyes

---

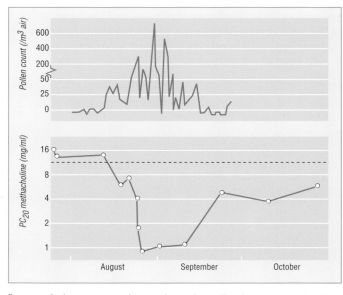

Increased airway responsiveness in patient allergic to ragweed pollen during ragweed season

response also develops after three hours; it peaks at 6-12 hours and may persist for 12-24 hours. Low molecular weight chemicals can provoke isolated late reactions.

The immediate asthmatic response is mediated by IgE dependent mast cell release of mediators such as histamine and leukotrienes. The late reaction is a manifestation of eosinophilic airway inflammation. Both are thought to be the outcome of a Th2 lymphocyte response to inhaled allergen.

The late, but not immediate, reaction is associated with the development of airway hyper-responsiveness, probably as a manifestation of the induced airway inflammation. The induced airway hyper-responsiveness occurs independently of the reduction in forced expiratory volume in one second and in airway calibre during the late reaction and can be sustained for several days after the forced expiratory volume has returned to normal. During the period of increased airway responsiveness the normal diurnal variation in airway calibre may be exaggerated, causing recurrent nocturnal asthma, and non-specific stimuli (such as exercise, cold air and smoke), as well as specific allergens to which the individual has developed specific IgE antibody, can provoke immediate asthmatic responses.

Allergen exposure and chronic asthma

Exposure to allergens induces late asthmatic responses and associated airway hyper-responsiveness. Airway hyper-responsiveness is an important determinant of immediate airway responses both to non-specific stimuli (such as exercise and cold air) and to exposure to specific allergens. By increasing non-specific airway responsiveness, allergen exposure can increase the development and persistence of chronic asthma.

Implications for treatment

This model has important implications for the management of asthma. Reducing allergen exposure at home or in the workplace will reduce not only the frequency of immediate asthmatic responses but also the severity of airway responsiveness and the capacity for allergens to provoke asthmatic responses. This is particularly important when a single "dominant" allergen is primarily responsible for the induction of asthma. Examples are occupational asthma and some cases of asthma caused by allergens in the home, such as house dust mite, cat, or cockroach, where avoidance measures have been shown to be effective.

Identification of allergens in the home and of allergens or chemicals encountered at work is therefore important when avoidance is practicable. In the home, pets are particularly relevant, and, with improved avoidance measures, identification of allergy to house dust mite is becoming more relevant.

In the workplace, accurate and early identification of the specific cause of allergic asthma (either allergen or chemical) to enable avoidance of further exposure is the cornerstone of management of occupational asthma.

The first graph is adapted with permission from Boulet et al (*J Allergy Clin Immunol* 1983;71:399-406), and the second is adapted with permission from Cockcroft et al (*Clin Allergy* 1997;7:503-73).

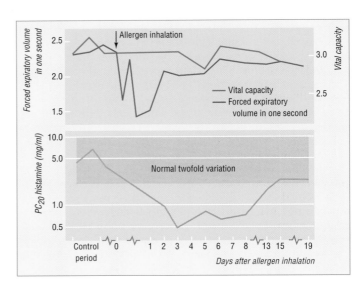

Increased airway responsiveness associated with late asthmatic reaction provoked by ragweed pollen

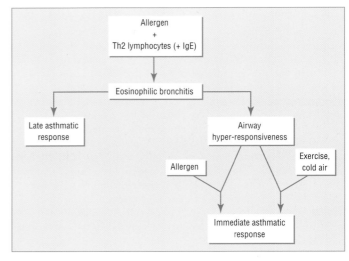

Allergen induction of airway inflammation and hyper-responsiveness permits provocation of immediate asthmatic responses by both allergens and non-specific factors, such as exercise and cold air

Criteria for diagnosing hypersensitivity induced occupational asthma

History
- Exposure to a sensitising agent
- Initial symptom free period of exposure (or employment)
- Improvement in severity of asthmatic symptoms during absences from work—eg, weekends or holidays—and progressive deterioration during periods at work

Objective evidence
- Serial peak flow measurements showing work related asthma
- Specific IgE (skin tests or in serum) to specific agent
- Reproducible late asthmatic response and increase in airway responsiveness provoked by inhalation test with specific agent in less than toxic concentrations*

*Inhalation tests should be undertaken only for medical purposes in a specialist centre when the diagnosis of occupational asthma remains uncertain after other investigations have been completed. Inhalation tests are not justifiable when undertaken solely for medicolegal purposes

9 Occupational asthma

Paul Cullinan

Definitions

Asthma is said to be occupational if it has been initiated by an agent inhaled at work. Classically, occupational asthma results from a Type I hypersensitivity response to an airborne allergen or hapten–protein conjugate. Where serological evidence of an immune response (the production of specific IgE antibodies to the causative agent) is available, demonstration of such a mechanism may be straightforward; it is more difficult with agents which do not readily provoke an identifiable antibody response — and in situations where there is a prior history of asthma. Patients whose pre-existing asthma is provoked by any of the very large number of workplace irritants are said to have work-related asthma. The distinction between 'occupational' and 'work-related' asthma may be difficult (and in some cases largely semantic), but it has important functional, economic and legal implications.

Because occupational asthma is primarily an immunological disease, it has a number of characteristic features which may be useful clinically: first, it occurs only in a proportion of those exposed to the causative agent(s), presumably reflecting genetic susceptibility. Second, its onset is not immediate but, because of the period required for sensitisation, generally several months or more after the start of a new occupation. Third, once occupational asthma has developed then symptoms may be provoked by very low intensity exposures to the initiating agent. The accompanying bronchial hyperresponsiveness may also mean that patients with established occupational asthma experience wheeze on exposure to a variety of non-specific respiratory irritants both at and away from work. This may be a source of some diagnostic confusion.

Causitive agents

Some 200–300 workplace agents have been demonstrated to be capable of inducing asthma. Happily, about a dozen only are responsible for the bulk of disease in the United Kingdom, and other similar industrialised countries. For convenience they are often categorised as being of 'high' or 'low' molecular weights. The former are generally of biological origin and act as complete allergens; they include, importantly, proteins excreted by laboratory animals, flour allergens, enzymes used in the food and detergent industries and proteins arising from natural rubber latex. Low-molecular-weight, or 'chemical' agents probably act as haptens, becoming allergenic after conjugation with one or more serum proteins. Important examples include diisocyanate hardening agents (especially those used in 'two-pack' polyurethane paints), colophony fume produced in electronic soldering and glutaraldehyde; although the frequency with which the last causes occupational asthma is controversial.

Frequency

A nationwide surveillance scheme in the United Kingdom (SWORD) reports about 2000 new cases of occupational asthma each year; this makes it the leading cause of

Occupations at high risk of occupational asthma	
Occupation	*Causative agent*
• Spray painting	• Diisocyanate hardening agents
• Laboratory animal research	• Urinary proteins
• Health care	• Latex, bone cement
• Electronic assembly	• Colophony (solder) fume
• Detergent powder manufacture	• Biological enzymes
• Baking	• Flour, enzymes
• Precious metal refining	• Complex platinum salts
• Plastics assembly	• Cyanoacrylate glues

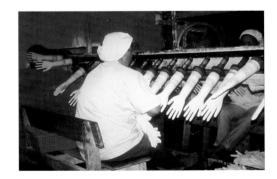

Latex glove manufacture

occupational respiratory disease in that country. Almost certainly the figure is an underestimate, perhaps by three-fold. Similar schemes operate, or are being set up, in other countries. Using crude denominator information, this figure equates to an overall annual incidence of about 20 cases per million working persons; naturally in some industrial settings the risk is very much higher. It is estimated that some 10% of laboratory animal workers or paint sprayers, for example, will develop asthma as a result of exposures encountered at work.

Studies based outside industry, in the general community, suggest that between 2 and 5% of all adult asthma may be attributed to occupational exposures; such studies do not readily differentiate asthma initiated, from that provoked, by work exposures.

Diagnosis

In many cases the patient with occupational asthma will recount an unmistakable history of wheeze which started after new employment (typically within two years) and which is worse at work and relieved during days off. Those whose disease is the result of exposure to a high-molecular-weight agent often report associated symptoms typical of an immune response to an airborne protein: rhinitis, itching and watering of the eyes and sometimes an urticarial rash. In other cases the relationship with work may be less clear. Where, for example, the clinical response is confined to a 'late-phase' asthmatic reaction then symptoms, confusingly, may be felt only after, rather than at work; night waking with wheeze or cough is a useful clue. Variable shift patterns, differences in day-to-day exposures within a job and pre-existing asthma may each complicate the pattern further. Particularly when confronted with a patient in a high-risk occupation, the clinician requires a low threshold for suspicion.

Patients with pre-existing atopic disease — hayfever, childhood asthma or eczema for example — are at an increased risk of developing occupational asthma to most high- (but not low-) molecular-weight agents. The disease is not, however, confined to those who are atopic and most atopic employees will not develop occupational asthma. For these reasons, 'atopy' is too crude a categorisation for the selection of potential employees into a workforce — even if such a process was considered desirable.

Investigations

A stepwise approach to confirming, or otherwise, a diagnosis of occupational asthma is useful:
1. Does this patient have asthma?
2. If so, is this related to his or her work?
3. If so, is the relationship causal?

Asthma — variable airflow limitation — can be verified in the usual ways. Crucially, it should be noted that clinic measurements of reversibility may be negative if the patient has not recently been exposed to the causative agent — has not been at work. Thus a normal FEV_1 with no response to a bronchodilator or a normal test for non-specific bronchial hyperreactivity does not rule out a diagnosis of occupational asthma. Most authorities advocate the use of serial peak flow measurements made both at home and at work, at least four times a day over a period of four or more weeks. With experienced readers, these become a very sensitive and specific tool for the diagnosis of work-related asthma.

Evidence of immunological sensitisation — the production of specific IgE antibodies assessed using skin prick tests or in serum — provides valuable supportive evidence. For most high-molecular-weight agents this is considered a wholly sensitive test (i.e. the absence of such antibodies effectively rules out a diagnosis of occupational asthma). It is generally

> **Stepwise approach to a diagnosis of occupational asthma:**
> 1 Does this patient have symptoms consistent with asthma?
> 2 Are symptoms temporally related to a new occupation; and with being at work?
> 3 Is there physiological confirmation of variable airflow limitation (asthma)?— serial measurements of peak flow at and away from work.
> 4 If appropriate, is there evidence of specific IgE production?
> 5 Is specific bronchial provocation testing required?

> **Indications for bronchial provacation testing**
> - Diagnostic uncertainty despite adequate prior investigation
> - Impracticability of serial peak flow measurements
> - Uncertainty about which of several potential agents may be implicated
>
> Note: provocation testing is not indicated solely for medicolegal purposes

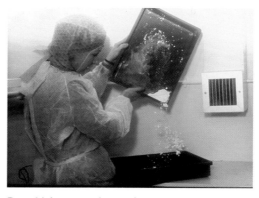

Bronchial provocation testing.

less helpful with low-molecular-weight agents, although there are some important exceptions. At present there are reliable techniques for detecting IgE antibodies to complex platinum salts and several acid anhydrides, but not to colophony fume or glutaraldehyde. Specific IgE antibodies to diisocyanate: human serum albumen conjugates are detected in about a third of patients with isocyanate-induced asthma, but when present are considered highly specific for a diagnosis of occupational asthma.

If doubt remains, then specific bronchial provocation testing — in a specialised centre — is indicated. This should be carried out under carefully regulated, placebo-controlled, single-blind conditions with experienced medical cover. By regular measurements of FEV_1 and bronchial reactivity following 'active' and 'inert' inhalations in an exposure chamber, a variety of typical asthmatic responses may be elicited. Provocation testing is generally considered the 'gold standard' diagnostic test for occupational asthma.

Management and outcome

Most patients with occupational asthma will improve when exposure to the causative agent ceases; either through adjustments within their job or, regrettably often, through a change in occupation. Patients with established occupational asthma generally find that their symptoms are protracted by vanishingly small exposures to the causative agent; for this reason the use of protective respiratory equipment at work may offer only a temporary respite. Inhaled steroids may alleviate — but rarely abolish — symptoms. There is good evidence that complete recovery from occupational asthma is less frequent in those who have continued to be exposed for long periods after the onset of their disease.

These facts should be explained to the patient in order to help them come to an informed decision about their employment; the guidance of the occupational physician, where there is one, should also be sought. Patients with occupational asthma are eligible to claim Industrial Injuries Disablement Benefit, the details of which (leaflet N1237 — 'If you have asthma because of your job') are available at any local office of the Department of Social Security (Benefits Agency).

Many patients with occupational asthma, particularly those with few professional qualifications, find considerable difficulties with future employment; false-positive diagnoses — the attribution of an 'occupational aetiology where one does not exist — may be disastrous in this respect.

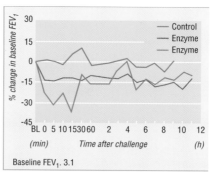

Baseline FEV_1. 3.1

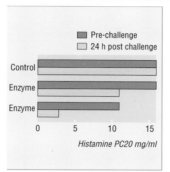

Detergent enzyme provocation testing

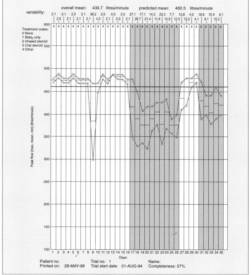

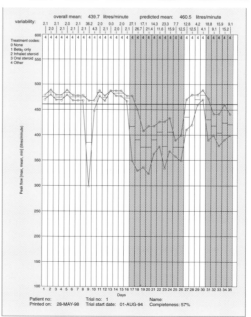

Example of serial peak flow measurements in a nurse with occupational asthma from latex. Days at work are shaded grey.

10 Avoiding exposure to indoor allergens

Ashley Woodcock, Adnan Custovic

The practice of avoiding exposure to allergens (allergen avoidance) for allergic diseases such as asthma is not a new idea. In the 16th century the Archbishop of St Andrews had a miraculous remission of his intractable asthma by getting rid of his feather bedding, and in 1927 Storm van Leeuwen created a "climate chamber" in Holland in an attempt to recreate the beneficial environment of high altitude sanatoriums. This article focuses on how to avoid indoor allergens in homes in temperate climates and the potential benefits for sensitised patients with atopic disorders.

Nowadays most people spend more than 90% of their lives indoors. Over the past 30 years, the home environment has changed enormously with the introduction of soft furnishings, fitted carpets, and central heating. Indoor ventilation has decreased—the rate at which indoor air is exchanged for fresh air is now 10 times lower than it was 30 years ago, with a considerable increase both in humidity and in concentrations of indoor pollutants and airborne allergens. As exposure to allergens is an important cause of symptoms in sensitised patients, reducing exposure should improve disease control. In spite of this, few patients in Britain with asthma, eczema, or perennial rhinitis, or any combination of these, are skin tested.

Characteristics of indoor allergens

The predominant indoor allergens in Britain are from mites, cats, and dogs, and they have dramatically different aerodynamic characteristics. Mite allergens are present on large particles in beds, soft furnishings, and carpets, which become airborne only after vigorous disturbance and settle quickly. In contrast, about 25% of cat and dog allergens are associated with small particles < 5 μm in diameter, which after disturbance remain airborne for prolonged periods. This in part explains the difference in clinical presentation between asthmatic people who are sensitive to mites and those sensitive to pets. Patients allergic to dust mite may be unaware of the relation between asthma and exposure to mites, as this is a predominantly low grade chronic exposure occurring overnight in bed. Patients allergic to cats or dogs may develop symptoms within minutes of entering a home with these animals or simply by stroking an animal, as a result of inhaling large amounts of easily respirable cat and dog allergen.

For symptoms to occur, atopic patients need to be exposed to allergens to which they are sensitised. Allergen avoidance should be recommended only to those symptomatic individuals who are sensitised on the basis of skin tests or specific serum IgE concentration.

Mites

Lessons from high altitude
At high altitude, low levels of humidity mean that mites cannot survive, and so mite allergen concentrations are low. Asthma control in mite sensitive patients moving to high altitude improves, although full improvement may take 6-12 months to achieve. The real challenge facing physicians in Britain is to create a low allergen environment in patients' homes that is sufficiently flexible to suit individual needs and at the same

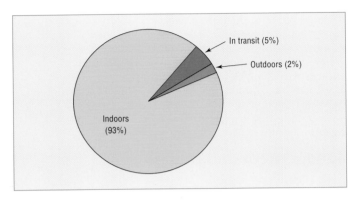

Amount of time Americans spend indoors, outdoors, and in transit

> **Few patients in Britain with asthma, eczema, or perennial rhinitis receive advice on appropriate avoidance measures**

___

Concentrations of indoor allergens
- The highest concentration of mite allergens is found in beds; patients spend 6-8 hours every night in close contact with their mattress, pillow, and bedding, so the reduction of exposure in the bedroom is critical
- Most exposure to pet allergens probably occurs in living areas other than the bedroom, and this must be taken into account when planning avoidance strategies
- In public areas—for example, cinemas and public transport—mite allergen levels are low, but exposure to airborne pet allergens can be substantial even in hospital outpatient areas
- Exposure to cockroach allergens may be important in schools and some high rise blocks of flats

___

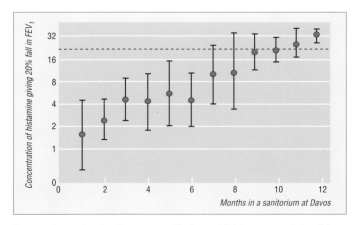

Progressive reduction in non-specific bronchial hyperreactivity (histamine) in 10 asthmatic children allergic to mites who moved from home to a mite free environment (a sanatorium in Davos, Switzerland)

time not prohibitively expensive. Many avoidance measures have been tested, but only a few have been subjected to randomised controlled trials.

Controlling concentrations of mite allergens

Bedrooms

The single most effective measure is to cover the mattress, pillows, and duvet with covers that are impermeable to mite allergens. These covers used to be made of plastic and were uncomfortable to sleep on. Now fabrics permeable to water vapour (either microporous or polyurethane coated) but also both impermeable to mite allergens and comfortable to sleep on are available. Allergen concentrations decrease by up to 100-fold after such covers are introduced.

All exposed bedding should be washed at 55°C. This kills mites and removes allergen; although the "cold" cycle (30°C) of laundry washing dramatically reduces allergen concentrations, most mites survive it. The covers should be wiped down at each change of bedding.

Buying a new mattress produces only a temporary benefit as reinfestation may occur within a few months from other reservoirs, such as carpets. Ideally, bedroom carpets should be replaced with sealed wooden or vinyl flooring, and the curtains should be hot washed regularly or replaced with wipeable blinds. In this way exposure to mite allergens in the bedroom at night can be virtually abolished. Substantial clinical benefit of effective mite avoidance has been shown in mite sensitised asthmatic patients and in patients with eczema or perennial rhinitis.

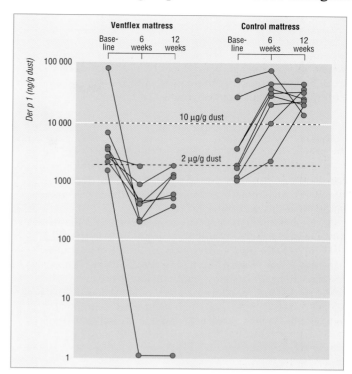

Approximate 100-fold reduction in concentrations of house dust mite allergen (Der p 1) on mattresses after introduction of covers that are impermeable to mite allergensd (Ventflex covers)

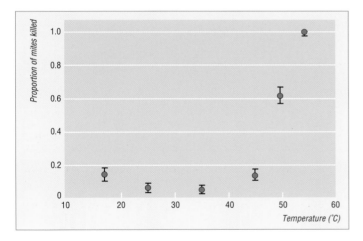

Proportion of mites killed at different washing temperatures

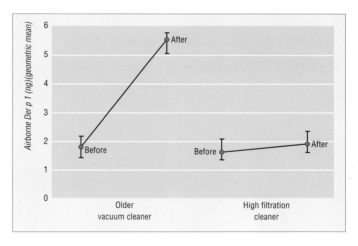

Comparision of older vacuum cleaner (with inadequate exhaust filtration) with high filtration cleaner, showing significantly increased concentrations of airborne house dust mite allergens (Der p 1) in older cleaners before and after vacuuming

Rest of the house

Intensive vacuum cleaning with high filtration cleaners reduces the size of the allergen reservoir, but no benefit has been established in a clinical trial. Older vacuum cleaners with inadequate exhaust filtration should be avoided as they provide one of the few ways to get large amounts of mite allergen airborne. Sensitised asthmatic patients who have to use a vacuum cleaner should use one with a built-in high efficiency particulate air filter and also use double thickness bags.

Killing mites with chemicals (acaricides) is feasible in the laboratory, but convincing evidence of clinical benefit is lacking. Mites can be killed in carpets either with steam or by freezing with liquid nitrogen, but both techniques are unlikely to produce sufficient benefits to warrant the huge effort required (in addition, regular treatment is necessary). Air filters and ionisers are of no clinical benefit as mite allergen does not stay airborne.

Actions for avoiding exposure to mite allergens in relation to asthma in Britain

Do help	May help	Do not help
Special bed covers (with or without cleaning)	Acaricides	
	Liquid	Air filters or ionisers
Removal of habitat (eg, carpet)	nitrogen	Ventilation systems
Moving to Switzerland	Tannic Acid	Dehumidifiers

A final alternative might be to reduce humidity to suppress the growth of mites. This has been attempted by the use of mechanical ventilation and with portable dehumidifiers. Neither of these techniques reduces humidity levels in typical British houses sufficiently to suppress mite growth, and allergen concentrations have not been shown to be reduced.

Pet allergens

Pet allergens are present in huge concentrations in houses with cats and dogs, but they are also transferred on clothing, so concentrations are detectable in homes without pets and in public buildings and transport.

For an asthmatic patient who owns a pet and is sensitised to the animal, the best way to reduce exposure is to get rid of the pet. This is rarely feasible as owners are usually very attached to their pets. Even after permanent removal of a cat or dog from the home, it may take many months before the reservoir allergen concentration returns to normal. So if patients do get rid of their pets they should not expect their symptoms to improve immediately—it may take 6-12 months for full benefit.

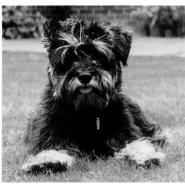

Milo: could you get rid of her?

If the pet remains in the home, advice can be given about methods that are known to reduce airborne pet allergens. The pet should be kept out of the bedroom and preferably outdoors or in a well ventilated area—for example, a kitchen. In homes with a pet, the concentration of airborne pet allergens will be considerable higher when the pet is actually in a room than when it is elsewhere in the house.

Ideally, carpets should be removed, as the concentration of pet allergens can be as much as 100 times higher in carpets than in polished floors. If carpets remain then regular cleaning with a high filtration cleaner is advised. Washing the animal thoroughly and as often as possible, combined with the use of a high efficiency particulate air filtration unit, is the best way to reduce allergens, but whether these practices are clinically effective is as yet unproved.

Allergen avoidance in primary prevention of atopic diseases

Sensitisation to allergens seems to be related to exposure to allergens in early life. The key question is whether early allergen avoidance can prevent allergic disease developing in the first place.

The innovative Isle of Wight study has examined the effect of avoiding mite allergens and certain foods from birth onwards on the development of atopy and asthma. This study used acaricides, and hence the reduction in the concentration of mite allergens was relatively modest. Even these minor

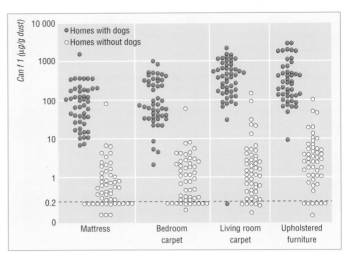

Distribution of dog allergen (Can f 1) in settled dust from four sampling sites in 100 homes in Manchester (50 with a dog, 50 without). Can f 1 was readily detectable in homes without dogs, but the levels were between 10-fold and 250-fold lower than in houses with dogs

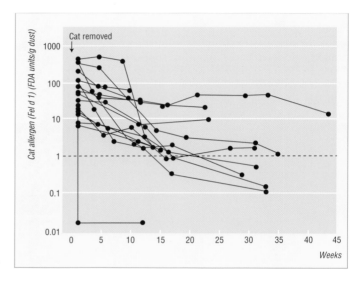

Effect on allergen concentrations a cat from a house

Avoiding cat and dog allergens

	Reduce airborne allergen	Gives clinical benefit
Removal of pet	✔	✔
Pet in situ:		
Wash pet	✔	?
Remove carpets	✔	?
High efficiency participate air filter	✔	?
Castrate male or get a female (cat)	✔	?

reductions, however, were associated with a reduction in sensitisation to mites, eczema, and episodic wheezing.

Several prospective cohorts of babies at high risk of atopy or asthma have been randomised to more effective protocols for avoiding exposure to mite allergens and are currently being studied. Population based studies are also being planned.

The future

Exposure to indoor allergens may have contributed to the observed increase in asthma prevalence. The important issue is whether asthma can be prevented by allergen avoidance in early life. Primary allergen avoidance is premature outside the context of a clinical trial but may be an important aspect of preventive therapy by the end of this century. Major changes in the domestic environment are likely over the next decade, with the removal of dust mite habitats—that is, a return to hard flooring—a reduction in indoor humidity, and the encasing of all bed and bedding with mite proof covers.

The following illustrations are reproduced or adapted with the permission of the publishers: the pie chart (Pope et al (*Indoor Allergens*, National Academy Press, 1993)); and the graphs showing results in children in Davos (Platts Mills et al (*J Allergy Clin Immunol* 1987;80:755-75)); allergen concentrations on mattresses (Owen S, et al (*Lancet* 1990;335:396-7)); mites killed during washing (McDonald et al (*J Allergy Clin Immunol* 1992;90:599-608)); concentrations of airborne house dust mite allergen in vacuum cleaners (Kalra S, et al (*Lancet* 1990;336:449)); distribution of dog allergen (Custovic A, et al (*Am J Respir Crit Care Med*—1997;155:94-8)); and effect on allergen concentrations by cat removal (Wood RA, et al (*J Allergy Clin Immunol* 1989;83:730-4)).

First steps in treating atopic diseases

- Diagnose disease by taking a history and by either performing skin testing or measuring specific serum IgE concentrations
- Minimise the impact of identified environmental risk factors such as mites, cats, and dogs
- Regard allergen avoidance as an integral part of the overall management of sensitised asthmatic patients

---

Further reading

- Platts Mills TAE, Vervloet D, Thomas WR, Aalberse RC, Chapman MD. Indoor allergens and asthma: report of the third international workshop. *J Allergy Clin Immunol* 1997;100(6):S1-24
- Custovic A, Simpson A, Chapman MD, Woodcock A. Allergen avoidance in the treatment of asthma and atopic disorders. *Thorax* 1998;53:63-72
- Collof MJ, Ayres J, Carswell F, Howarth PH, Merrett TG, Mitchell EB, et al. The control of allergens of dust mites and domestic pets: a position paper. *Clin Exp Allergy* 1992;22(suppl 2):1-28
- Pope AM, Patterson R, Burge H, eds. *Indoor allergens—assessing and controlling adverse health effects*. Washington, DC: National Academy Press, 1993

11 Allergy and the skin. I—Urticaria

Malcolm W Greaves, Ruth A Sabroe

Acute urticaria

Episodes of acute urticaria are common. Causes include type 1 hypersensitivity reactions to certain foods and drugs, including blood products. In up to 50% of cases a cause is not identified. The involvement of a particular food allergen can be confirmed by the radioallergosorbent test (RAST) and skin prick tests. Allergy to latex usually manifests as contact urticaria or with systemic symptoms but rarely presents with generalised urticaria. As with suspected reactions to peanuts it is recommended that tests for latex allergy be done in a hospital setting as severe systemic reactions may occur. Management of acute urticaria includes avoidance of the causative agent and treatment with H_1 antihistamines. A short course of prednisolone can be given for severe episodes of urticaria unresponsive to antihistamines.

Causes of acute urticaria

- Idiopathic origin
- Food: fruits (for example, strawberries), seafood, nuts, dairy products, spices, tea, chocolate
- Drugs: antibiotics (for example, penicillin) and sulphonamides; aspirin and non steroidal anti inflammatory drugs; morphine and codeine
- Blood products
- Viral infections and febrile illnesses
- Radio contrast media
- Wasp or bee stings

Chronic urticaria

Chronic urticaria is conventionally defined as the occurrence of daily or almost daily widespread itchy weals for at least six weeks. It occurs in at least 0.1% of the population and is much more troublesome than acute urticaria. Recent studies using an internationally recognised quality of life questionnaire, the Nottingham health profile, have highlighted the serious disability of patients with chronic urticaria, including loss of sleep and energy, social isolation, altered emotional reactions, and difficulties in aspects of daily living. The disability is of the same order as that experienced by patients with severe chronic ischaemic heart disease.

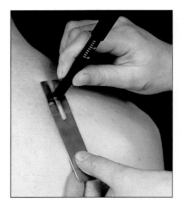
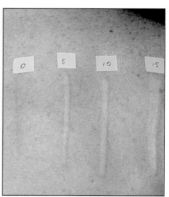

Dermographism induced with a calibrated, spring loaded dermographometer

Physical urticarias

The first step is to identify patients with physical urticarias. These are patients in whom wealing and itching is provoked at the sites of a physical stimulus—such as stroking the skin (dermographism), cooling the skin (cold urticaria), or sun exposure (solar urticaria). Cholinergic urticaria, a widespread transitory pruritic rash following exercise, emotion, or heat, also falls into this category.

Once these physical urticarias have been identified and the diagnosis confirmed if necessary by challenge testing, further investigation is unrewarding, and they are best treated symptomatically by avoidance and with antihistamines.

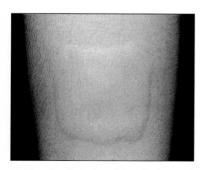

Cold urticaria induced by placing an ice cube on the skin for 5 minutes

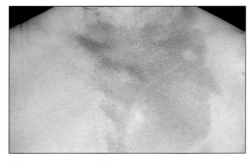

Solar urticaria, which can be induced by irradiation of the skin with a solar simulator

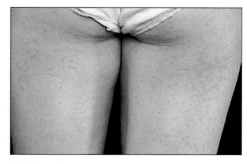

Cholinergic urticaria induced by brisk exercise

Physical urticarias frequently coexist with chronic "idio-pathic" urticaria (referred to in the rest of the article as chronic urticaria). In these cases management will depend on whether the physical urticaria or the chronic urticaria is the major contributor to the patient's disability.

Angio-oedema

Defined as deep mucocutaneous swellings, angio-oedema occurs concurrently with ordinary urticarial weals in about half of patients with chronic urticaria. Hereditary angio-oedema is a rare condition caused by an autosomal dominant inherited defect of the inhibitor of the first component of the complement cascade. Urticarial weals are not strictly a feature of hereditary angio-oedema, but if doubt exists, a normal value for the serum complement component C4 in between attacks effectively excludes this diagnosis in almost all cases.

Urticarial vasculitis

It is all too easy to overlook the occasional patient with urticarial vasculitis. The clinical picture of urticarial vasculitis may be distinctive, but more often the morphology of the weals resembles that of chronic urticaria and the only clinical clue is the duration of individual weals, which invariably persist for more than 24 hours. Confirmation of the diagnosis by a skin biopsy to show histological evidence of vasculitis is important because these patients need to be fully investigated for evidence of lupus erythematosus or other autoimmune connective tissue disease, and of renal or other internal organ involvement. They also usually require additional treatment measures—for example, dapsone, colchicine, or occasionally oral steroids.

Pathogenesis

The weals in chronic urticaria are caused by a local increase in cutaneous vascular permeability, mainly in the postcapillary venules. This, and the associated erythema and itching, is evoked by pharmacological mediators released from mast cells in the skin. Histamine, stored in the granules of mast cells and secreted as a result of degranulation, is the principal mediator; this is evident from the symptomatic relief afforded by H_1 antihistamines. Experimental wealing due to intracutaneous injection of histamine is short lived, lasting minutes rather than hours. In contrast, individual urticarial weals last 12 or more hours. This is due to the actions of additional mediators, some of which are probably also derived from the mast cells. There are some similarities between the histopathological appear-ances of urticarial weals and those of the late phase response. This may suggest the additional participation of basophil leucocytes that contain histamine.

Causes and investigation

Until recently the cause of chronic urticaria was unknown in nearly all cases. Today we still do not know the aetiology in many, but subsets of chronic urticaria can now be defined in which the cause can be identified, with important conse-quences for treatment.

Causes listed in most textbooks include infestations, candidiasis, and internal malignancy, although in practice none of these can be convincingly incriminated. A recent spate of reports have associated *Helicobacter pylori* and hepatitis C infection with chronic urticaria, but the evidence is not robust.

Chronic urticaria can occasionally be confirmed to be due to a specific food additive. Reproducible placebo controlled oral challenge testing is essential for diagnosis; failure to appreciate this probably accounts for the frequency with which food additives have been implicated in chronic urticaria in some study series. Challenge testing should be blind challenge by

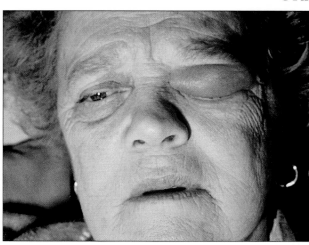

Mucocutaneous angio-oedema

Features suggestive of urticarial vasculitis

Clinical
- Duration of weals >24 hours
- Weals painful rather than itchy
- Residual purpura, bruising, or pigmentary change
- Prominent systemic features (eg, fever, nephritis, arthralgia)
- Poor response to antihistamines

Laboratory
- High erythrocyte sedimentation rate and raised concentrations of acute phase proteins

Histopathology
- Venular endothelial cell swelling and disruption
- Leucocyte invasion of venular endothelium
- Extravasation of red cells
- Leucocytoclasia (neutrophil nuclear dust)
- Fibrin deposition

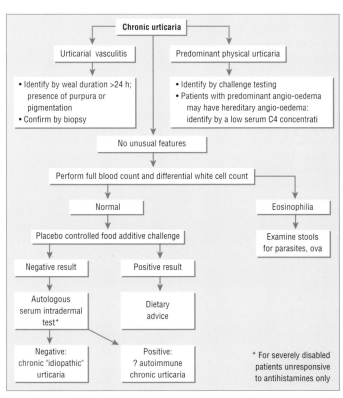

Investigation of chronic urticaria

numbered capsules containing the food additives suspected of being implicated (details from authors on request). A substantiated positive result should prompt appropriate dietetic advice. In our practice, food additives are confirmed as the cause in only about 0.6-0.8% of patients with chronic urticaria. Exclusion diets are usually unhelpful: the results are difficult to interpret and even misleading; compliance is poor; and the administration of such diets unwieldy and prolonged.

Autoimmune chronic urticaria

In about 50-60% of patients with chronic urticaria the weals are caused by circulating histamine releasing factors. In half of these the histamine releasing activity has been proved to be due to IgG autoantibodies directed against epitopes expressed on the extracellular portion of the α subunit of the high affinity IgE receptor (FCϵRIα), which is located on the outer surface of all mast cells and basophil leucocytes. This autoantibody, which is of isotype IgG_1 or IgG_3, is functional because it releases histamine from mast cells or basophils in vitro and causes wealing upon intradermal injection in humans in vivo. Anti-FCϵRI autoantibodies cross link α subunits of adjacent FCϵRI, thereby triggering release of histamine. In a very small minority of such patients the autoantibody has proved to be an IgG anti-IgE autoantibody, but the result seems to be the same.

The clinical presentation of autoimmune urticaria seems to be indistinguishable from that of autoantibody-negative chronic urticaria. Although autoimmune urticaria can currently be identified only in specialist units, it is very important for the management of these patients that their autoantibodies are identified. Treatment of patients with autoimmune urticaria by plasmapheresis or intravenous immunoglobulin infusions has brought about remissions in patients who were previously severely affected, badly disabled, and resistant to treatment.

Natural course

Characteristically, chronic urticaria pursues a course of remission and relapse, relapses being triggered by intercurrent infections, stress, drugs (especially aspirin and angiotensin converting enzyme inhibitors), and the menstrual cycle. It has been estimated that about 50% of patients presenting with a history of chronic urticaria of at least 3 months' duration will still have the condition three years later.

Treatment

Patients should be advised to avoid factors that trigger relapses, especially non-steroidal anti-inflammatory drugs. As weals tend to occur at sites of local pressure, tightly fitting clothes, belts, and shoes should be avoided. Itching is exacerbated by warmth, and therefore a cool ambient temperature, especially in the bedroom, is helpful and may prevent insomnia.

Treatment with 1% menthol in aqueous cream has been proved to suppress histamine induced itching, and many patients find it helpful. Mucocutaneous angio-oedema can be treated by two to three puffs of an aqueous 2% ephedrine spray. Unlike hereditary or acute allergic angio-oedema, angio-oedema in association with chronic urticaria is rarely life threatening, although it can be very unpleasant and frightening.

Antihistamines are still the mainstay of treatment of chronic urticaria, although they tend to be more effective in suppressing itching than wealing. Before antihistamines are chosen, the timing of administration must be considered. Patients frequently experience flare ups at certain times of the day—for example, after lunch or in the early evening. The course of action of the antihistamine chosen must ensure cover of these diurnal peaks. Low sedation H_1 antihistamines, such as cetirizine, fexofenidine and loratadine daily, are useful for daytime treatment. Cetirizine 10mg daily is also useful,

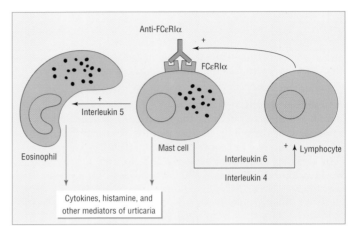

Probable pathogenesis of wealing in autoimmune (anti-FCϵRI) chronic urticaria. Activation of cutaneous mast cells by anti-FCϵRIα auto-antibodies leads to release of proinflammatory mediators and also to activation of eosinophils (via interleukin 5) and immunoglobulin-synthesising B lymphocytes (via interleukin 4 and interleukin 6)

Treatment of chronic idiopathic urticaria
- Avoidance of precipitating or exacerbating factors
  Food additives, alcohol, hot environment, stress
  Aspirin and non-steroidal anti-inflammatory drugs, codeine and morphine
  Angiotensin converting enzyme inhibitors if there is angio-oedema
- Topical treatments
  Tepid shower
  1% menthol in aqueous cream
  2% ephedrine spray for oral angio-oedema
- H_1 antihistamines (with or without H_2 antihistamines) or doxepin
- Short reducing course of prednisolone
- Specialist treatments
  Cyclosporin A
  Intravenous immunoglobulins
  Plasmapheresis

especially if there is associated delayed pressure urticaria, against which it seems to have a selective action. Care must be taken not to administer terfenadine or astemizole with cytochrome P-450 inhibitors including doxepin, imidazole antifungals and macrolide antibiotics, to avoid cardiac arrhythmic complications. Doxepin is useful as a single night time 25mg dose in patients who experience nocturnal disease activity especially when associated with anxiety or depression. A combination of cetirizine in the morning and doxepin in the late evening affords symptomatic relief, even in severely affected patients with recalcitrant urticaria. Although combinations of H_2 and H_1 antihistamines have been shown to be more effective than either class of antihistamine alone in some studies, the gain is too small to be clinically useful.

Systemic steroids are not indicated in chronic urticaria owing to the substantial doses required, the development of tolerance, and frequency of chronic steroid toxicity. In exceptional circumstances, however, short tapering courses of prednisolone have a place when rapid control over a limited period is required.

There have been several reports of the value of $\beta2$ adrenergics (for example, terbutaline), calcium channel antagonists (for example, nifedipine), and anabolic steroids (for example, stanazolol) in the management of chronic urticaria. These studies lack underpinning by controlled trial data and are unconvincing.

Immunosuppressive treatment in autoantibody (anti-$FC\epsilon RI\alpha$)-positive chronic urticaria as discussed above, as well as cyclosporin, may be dramatically beneficial in selected patients, but these treatments should be provided by specialised centres.

No antihistamines are safe in pregnancy, but if antihistamines have to be administered to control chronic urticaria, chlorpheniramine is advised as it has the best safety record

Further reading

- Greaves MW. Chronic urticaria. *N Engl J Med* 1995;332:1767-72
- Hide M, Francis DM, Grattan CEH, Hakimi J, Kochan JP, Greaves MW. Autoantibodies against the high-affinity IgE receptor as a cause of histamine release in chronic urticaria. *N Engl J Med* 1993;328:1599-604
- Sabroe RA, Greaves MW. The pathogenesis of chronic idiopathic urticaria. *Arch Dermatol* 1996;23:735-40
- O'Donnell BF, Black AK. Urticarial vasculitis. *Int Angiol* 1995;14:166-74
- Champion RH, Roberts SOB, Carpenter RG, Roger JH. Urticaria and angioedema: a review of 554 patients. *Br J Dermatol* 1969;81:588-97

St John's Institute of Dermatology provided the first five photographs in the article. The photograph showing mucocutaneous angio-oedema is published with permission of the patient, whose grandson, Robert Payne, provided the photograph.

12 Allergy and the skin. II—Contact and atopic eczema

P S Friedmann

Allergic contact eczema

Eczema is characterised by erythema, pruritus, vesiculation, and, in more chronic forms, scaly desquamation. Contact eczema may be due to chemically induced irritation or allergic sensitisation. Allergic contact eczema is a cell mediated (delayed type) hypersensitivity reaction to environmental chemical "sensitisers." Hence, it occurs at body sites that make physical contact with the eliciting sensitiser. The term dermatitis is often used for eczema caused by exogenous agents.

Prevalence and aetiology
In the working population of Western countries, contact eczema (both irritant and allergic) accounts for 85-90% of all occupational skin disease. Hand eczema has been estimated to affect 2-6.5% of all populations in Western countries.

The development of allergic reactions to exogenous substances seems to be the result of the intrinsic "sensitising potency" of the compound and various host factors that determine susceptibility. Small molecular chemicals vary in their potential to induce allergic sensitivity: primula can sensitise most people, nickel sensitises 10-20% of women, while many other agents sensitise a smaller minority. The sensitising potency of a chemical is thought to be related to its chemical reactivity and ability to bind to proteins, which act as "carriers," facilitating the presentation of the substance to the immune system. Host susceptibility is related to as yet uncharacterised genetic factors, which include variation in metabolic pathways that handle exogenous chemicals.

Mechanisms
When skin sensitisers penetrate the epidermis, they are taken up by Langerhans' cells—bone marrow-derived members of the macrophage family that function as "professional antigen presenting cells." The Langerhans' cells leave the epidermis and migrate to the regional lymph nodes, where they enter the paracortical areas, the home of naive T lymphocytes. Probably while en route to the lymph node, the Langerhans' cells process the sensitiser so it is physically associated with the HLA-DR molecules on the cell surface. In the node, the Langerhans' cells "present" the sensitiser to T lymphocytes of the immune system. If T cells with the appropriate specific receptor recognise the complex of sensitiser and HLA-DR, they proliferate to establish "immunological memory." The memory T cells that mediate allergic contact eczema are of the Th1 subtype, characterised by the production of interleukin 2 and interferon gamma. The induction of sensitisation and establishment of immunological memory takes 8-14 days. Should re-exposure to the sensitiser occur, Langerhans' cells carry it down into the dermis, where they present it to memory T cells travelling through the tissues. These are activated to release cytokines (including interferon gamma) that attract other cells and activate vascular responses, resulting in the characteristic inflammation of contact eczema.

Dierential diagnosis
Allergic contact eczema must be distinguished from irritant contact eczema. Clinically the two may be indistinguishable, but irritant eczema usually occurs on the hands. It is the result

Distribution of allergic contact eczema
- Nickel sensitivity involves ears, skin under buckles, and often the hands; accidental spread from hands can involve the face
- Hair products (for example, dyes, perms, and setting agents) often affect the face, neck, and ears
- Clothing dyes in socks and shoe leather often affect the feet
- Ingredients in drugs used around leg ulcers often induce a dermatitis of the leg

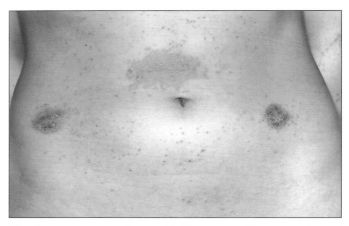

Allergic contact eczema due to nickel in studs and buttons on jeans

Clinical presentation
- After re-exposure to a sensitiser, at sites of skin contact with the offending agent, an itchy erythematous rash starts to develop within 6-12 hours
- The reaction progresses and reaches a peak between 48 and 72 hours after contact
- Sensitivity may range from weak to strong
- Strongly sensitised people may need very little contact to evoke an acute, weeping eczematous reaction
- Nickel in keys, money, or clothing studs can be eluted by minimal perspiration through several layers of clothes

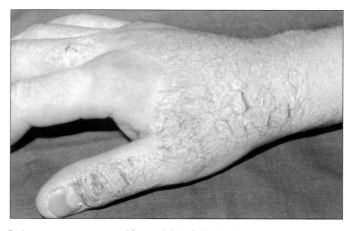

Irritant contact eczema (dermatitis) of the hand

of repeated "insult" to the skin with caustic, irritant, or detergent substances. Photoallergic eczema occurs on light exposed areas—face, nape of neck, and backs of hands. It is usually a response to photosensitisation by ingested drugs such as thiazide diuretics or quinine.

Management

The causal agent should be identified by epicutaneous patch tests. Contact allergy can be induced by a huge range of substances encountered daily. Sometimes the history of flare ups after contact with something is sufficient to permit reasonably confident identification. Often a short list of possible culprits can be arrived at. Definitive proof of causal significance, however, requires patch testing. This is normally performed in dermatology clinics with the requisite expertise and range of test materials.

The patient should then be advised to avoid the causal agent.

Treatment will vary:
● Acute weeping eczema should be "dried" by soaking with potassium permanganate (1/10 000) daily for four to five days;
● Anti-inflammatory steroids of category 3 or 4 (category 1 is the weakest, 4 the strongest—see *British National Formulary*) during the acute phase;
● Systemic steroids may be required for severe cases;
● For irritant hand eczema, avoiding contact with soaps, detergents, and solvents, together with generous use of greasy emollients, is vital.

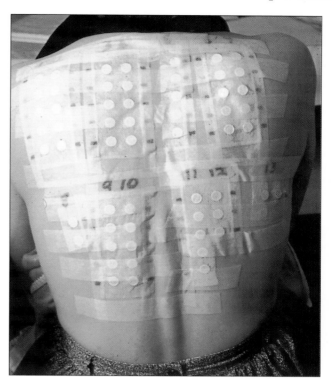

Patch testing for diagnosing causal sensitiser in allergic contact eczema

Atopic eczema

Definition

The atopic state is a genetically determined capacity to make IgE class antibodies to antigens that enter the body via mucosal surfaces. This is associated with allergies of the immediate type and the clinical syndromes of rhinitis asthma or atopic eczema, alone or in combination.

Prevalence

For unclear reasons the prevalence of atopic diseases, including eczema, has risen steadily over the past 30 years. There are many estimates of the prevalence of atopic eczema in children in different countries. For children aged up to 12 years these range from 12-26%.

With increasing age the prevalence falls: 65% of atopic eczema presents before the age of 6 months, and 80% in the first year of life.

Aetiology

In atopic individuals, responses to common allergens result in the generation of helper T lymphocytes of the so called Th2-type in preference to those of Th1-type.

Th2 cells produce mainly interleukins 4 and 5, which regulate IgE production, mast cells, and eosinophils. Th1 cells produce mainly interleukin 2 and interferon gamma. Although several potentially important genes are receiving attention, they seem more connected with the formation of IgE than with the clinical syndrome.

It is completely unknown what determines whether the clinical manifestations in any individual will involve the lungs, nose, or skin.

Clinical presentation

Atopic eczema most commonly begins in infancy. The rash of erythematous areas comprises tiny papules, sometimes with an

Pathogenesis

● Eczema is triggered or exacerbated by interactions between a genetic predisposition and environmental factors
● These include environmental allergens (house dust mites, animal furs, and pollens), microbes (such as staphylococci), environmental pollutants, and climatic and emotional factors
● Skin challenge with allergens elicits both immediate and delayed responses
● The evidence suggests that atopic eczema is an allergic reaction mediated by T lymphocytes of both Th1-types and Th2-types
● Although IgE may participate during antigen presentation and by mediation of immediate-type hypersensitivity responses, the eczema is probably not related to histamine or mast cell products

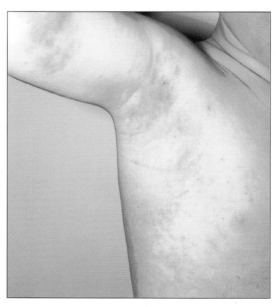

Typical atopic eczema in child

urticaria-like component. They may join to form confluent red sheets. In infants atopic eczema commonly affects the whole body including the head and face. On the limbs predominantly extensor surfaces are affected.

Once the baby begins to crawl, the eczema tends to localise to extensor surfaces of the hands, wrists, knees, and ankles. These changes in distribution are probably related to changes in exposure or contact with exogenous triggers, including friction from dusty floor surfaces. Once the toddling and upright stage is reached, the eczema moves to flexural sites such as popliteal and antecubital fossae. The severity may range from mild (usually of limited extent) to severe, with extensive, angry inflammation on most of the body.

> Acute exacerbations may be weepy and crusted—this usually signifies superinfection with staphylococci. Chronic excoriated lesions are often thickened and lichenified

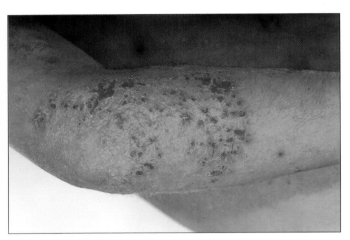

Discoid pattern of atopic eczema

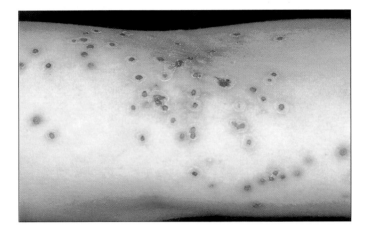

Eczema herpeticum (ulcers are of similar shape and size)

Complications

Immune resistance to several microbial pathogens is reduced in individuals with atopic eczema. Thus both viral warts and molluscum contagiosum can be numerous and slow to clear. Eczema herpeticum is infection with herpes simplex viruses, which may be extensive and aggressive.

> The key physical sign of eczema herpeticum is blisters, pustules, or erosions of a rather uniform size and appearance

Management

Drug treatment

The basis of direct treatment is to suppress the symptoms and control or prevent complications.

Atopic eczema is readily irritated by soaps, so their avoidance and use of emollients as soap substitutes is important.

Anti-inflammatory topical steroids are the mainstay of treatment. In children, when the eczema is very active, stronger steroids such as betamethasone valerate (1/4 strength) may be required. Normally, clobetasone or mometasone may be adequate for treating areas other than the face; 1% hydrocortisone is the main steroid for the face. In adults undiluted category 3 steroids may be required for flare ups. Dilutions and weaker steroids are used for regular maintenance.

Acute flares are often induced by staphylococcal super-infection. Systemic antibiotics (flucloxacillin or erythromycin) should be used. If chronic or repeated infective episodes occur, use of a topical steroid and antibiotic, or antiseptic mixtures, can help.

Although antihistamines are often used to relieve itch, histamine is not the main, responsible mediator. Hence antihistamines are not very effective, and usually the older sedative types—such as trimeprazine, hydroxyzine, and chlorpheniramine—seem more effective than the modern non-sedative varieties.

Treatment of atopic eczema

- Emollients as soap substitutes
- Oils, creams, and ointments
- Topical steroids to suppress inflammation
- Antibiotics
- Antihistamines—sedative varieties
- Bandages— "wet dressings" or impregnated bandages

Use of topical steroids for treating atopic eczema

	Adults	Children
When severe	Category 3 to body; category 2 to face	Diluted category 3 to body; category 2 to face
Routine	Category 2 or diluted category 3 to body; category 1 or 2 to face	Category 1 or 2 to body; category 1 (hydrocortisone) to face

Bandages and dressings
In infants and children the "wet bandage" technique can provide great symptomatic relief. A double layer of medium grade tubular cotton bandage (Tubifast, Seton) is applied over a layer of emollient or sometimes over a weak topical steroid. The inner layer of bandage is moistened with warm water. The dressing can be applied to limbs and even the trunk. For very lichenified or excoriated eczema, various bandages impregnated with antiseptics (Ichthopaste, Smith and Nephew, or Quinaband, Seton) or zinc oxide (Viscopaste, Smith and Nephew) can be used to occlude the area; a weak steroid and antiseptic mixture is usually applied underneath.

Second line treatment
Systemic corticosteroids should be used very seldom. Atopic eczema virtually always flares rapidly on dose reduction. Ultraviolet light (UVB) and photochemotherapy with a psoralen and long wavelength ultraviolet irradiation (UVA; PUVA) may be used in older children and adults.

Third line treatment
When second line treatment fails or is not suitable, various further treatment options are available (see box).

Allergen avoidance
The role of allergen avoidance should be considered for all patients with atopic eczema. Avoidance or elimination of house dust mite allergens can be beneficial for many people with confirmed mite sensitivity who have severe atopic eczema. The main study to show this looked at children aged over 6 years and adults. The most important measures are encasing the mattress in a dust proof bag, and washing the duvets and pillows every three months; washes should be hotter than 55°C to kill mites and denature antigens. Removal of fitted carpets in the bedroom should be recommended. Reducing upholstered furnishings and regular use of a modern cylinder or upright vacuum cleaner fitted with an adequate filter seem sensible precautions.

Foods are often suspected as being provoking factors in babies, but reliable identification of relevant foods is difficult and often impossible. Hence regimens avoiding dairy or other suspected foods are often disappointing, and if no clear benefit is obtained they should not be maintained for longer than four weeks. In small children such diets are difficult to implement, and the help of a dietician is necessary.

The photograph showing dermatitis of the hand is reproduced with the permission of Gower Medical Publishing. The data in the graph are adapted from Tan et al (*Lancet* 1996;347:15-8).

Third line treatment of atopic eczema
- Cyclosporin A can be highly beneficial in severe atopic eczema
- Great care must be taken in monitoring renal function, and treatment courses should be restricted to 8-12 weeks
- In adults with severe and chronic atopic eczema, azathioprine may be used for longer term maintenance
- Haematological and hepatic function must be monitored carefully

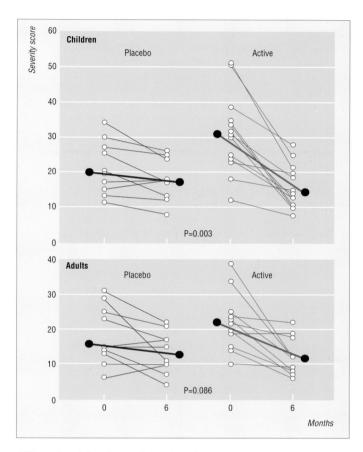

Effect of avoiding house dust mite allergens on severity of atopic aczema. Individual scores before and after 6 months' avoidance are connected by fine lines. Solid lines represent median scores for each group

Further reading
- Williams HC. Is the prevalence of atopic dermatitis increasing? *Clin Exp Dermatol* 1992;17:385-91
- Cooper KD. Atopic dermatitis: recent trends in pathogenesis and therapy. *J Invest Dermatol* 1994;102:128-37
- Friedmann PS, Tan BB, Musaba E, Strickland I. Pathogenesis and management of atopic dermatitis. *Clin Exp Allergy* 1995;25:799-806
- Tan BB, Weald D, Strickland I, Friedmann PS. Double blind controlled trial of house dust-mite allergen avoidance on atopic dermatitis. *Lancet* 1996;347:15-8
- Friedmann PS. Clinical aspects of allergic contact dermatitis. In: Kimber I, Maurer T, eds. *Toxicology of contact hypersensitivity*. London: Taylor and Francis, 1996:26-56

13 Food allergy

Carsten Bindslev-Jensen

The public perceives food allergy differently from doctors—especially in relation to its symptoms and prevalence. In controlled scientific studies a low prevalence of food allergy has been found in British and Dutch adults, whereas the percentage of people perceiving their illness as being food dependent is much higher. The prevalence in adults, confirmed by double blind, placebo controlled food challenge, has been estimated to be 1.4%. This is in contrast to findings in children, in whom the overall prevalence of IgE mediated food allergies is 5-7%.

Definitions

Adverse reactions to foods may be classified as due to either true food allergy or non-allergic food intolerance. In contrast, food aversion refers to symptoms that are often non-specific and unconfirmed by double blind, placebo controlled food challenge.

A true food allergy is a disorder in which ingestion of a small amount of food elicits an abnormal immunologically mediated clinical response. Food may cause allergic reactions by several mechanisms. The classic type I, IgE mediated reaction is the most thoroughly studied and potentially important in view of the risk of life threatening reactions in some people. Evidence is increasing, however, for an important role for delayed reactions (classic type IV mediated reactions). For example, eczema in children may be exacerbated by milk ingestion, and a small proportion of adults with severe contact dermatitis due to nickel may react to nickel in their diet.

Non-allergic food intolerance may be due to pharmacological, metabolic, and toxic causes. Pharmacological causes may provoke anaphylactoid reactions, flushing, hypotension, and urticaria. This can happen with foods with a high histamine content (for example, scombroid poisoning due to ingestion of brown oily fish (mackerel, tuna, etc) that has gone off). Tyramine in cheese or red wine may provoke or exacerbate migraine. Monosodium glutamate may provoke flushing, headache, and abdominal symptoms (the Chinese restaurant syndrome). Lactase deficiency in young children is an example of non-allergic food intolerance due to a metabolic cause, and it manifests as abdominal symptoms and chronic diarrhoea after ingestion of milk. Toxic reactions to foods may be due to contamination of food by chemicals or bacterial toxins.

Much overlooked is the harmless, non-immunologically mediated, immediate perioral flare reaction (non-immunological contact urticaria) to, for example, benzoic acid from citrus fruits in children (especially those with atopic dermatitis). Parents and doctors may misinterpret this response in a child as an allergy and unnecessarily stop the child from eating citrus fruits. Food additives and colourings may elicit an acute flare up reaction of urticaria and, more rarely, gastrointestinal symptoms, with or without exacerbation of urticaria, asthma, or rhinitis. Additives include benzoates, salicylates, sulphites, and tartrazine and other colourings. The diagnosis of these reactions should be suspected in patients who develop symptoms on exposure to foods that contain preservatives—for example, meat pies, sausages and other preserved meats, dried fruits that contain sulphite, and many commercially tinned and bottled foods. Preservatives may also

Prevalence (%) of adverse reactions to foods in adults*

Town	Perceived prevalence in adults	Confirmed prevalence†
High Wycombe	20.4	1.4

*Data from Young et al (*Lancet* 1994;1127–30).
†With double blind, placebo controlled fodd challenge

Types of adverse reactions to foods
- Food allergy due to IgE mediated mechanism (Coombs' classification, type I)
- Food allergy not involving IgE, in which other immunological mechanisms are implicated (for example, type IV)
- Non-allergic food intolerance (for example, pharmocological, metabolic, or toxic reactions to foods)
- Food aversion (symptoms are often non-specific and unconfirmed by blinded food challenge)

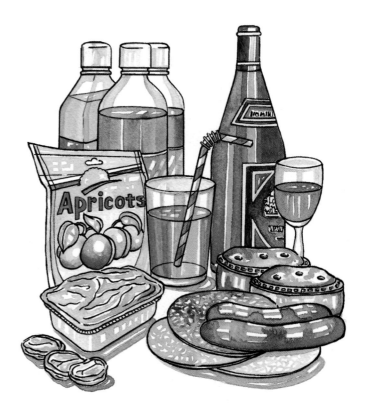

Common products containing preservatives

be sprayed on to salads to maintain freshness and are commonly present in alcoholic drinks and coloured fruit drinks. There are no diagnostic tests for reactions to preservatives or colourings. Diagnosis depends on suspicion and the use of elimination diets or blinded challenges with capsules containing preservatives and placebo capsules, or both of these approaches.

> "One man's meat is another man's poison"

Symptoms and signs of adverse reactions to foods

Patients with true IgE mediated food reactions generally identify either one or a limited number of specific foods that provoke symptoms, usually within minutes. A characteristic feature is the oral allergy syndrome—itching and swelling in the mouth and oropharynx followed, on further intake, by concomitant symptoms and signs from two or more of the following organ systems (the gastrointestinal tract, skin, and respiratory system). Life threatening reactions may include exacerbation of asthma, laryngeal oedema, and anaphylaxis with cardiovascular collapse.

Factors suggesting classic IgE mediated food allergy

- Specific food(s) can be identified
- Timing of symptoms is closely associated with food intake
- Symptoms are typical and involve more than one organ (for example, oral itching or swelling, nausea, vomiting, abdominal pain, diarrhoea, asthma, rhinitis, urticaria, angio-oedema, anaphylaxis)
- Patient has a personal or family history of other atopic disorders

Offending foods

Many foods have been claimed to cause allergy, but controlled studies show that a limited number of foods are responsible for the vast majority of cases. Common allergenic foods include milk, eggs, and peanuts in children; and fish, shellfish, nuts (especially peanuts), and fruit in adults. When clinically insignificant cross reactions are excluded, most patients react clinically to a few foods only. Food allergy may also result from exposure to food in the workplace.

Common foods provoking food allergy

Food	Cross reacting foods
Cows' milk	Mares' milk, goats' milk, ewes' milk
Hens' eggs	Eggs from other birds
Cod	Mackerel, herring, plaice, etc
Shrimps	Other crustaceans
Peanuts	Soy beans,* green beans,* green peas*
Soy beans	See above
Wheat	Other grains, most often rye
Additives	Mostly unknown (both synthetic and naturally occurring)

Patients allergic to pollen may have cross reactions with hazelnuts, green apples, peaches, almonds, kiwis, tomatoes, and potatoes* (birch pollen) or wheat,* rye,* and corn* (grass pollen)

*Without clinically significant serological cross reaction

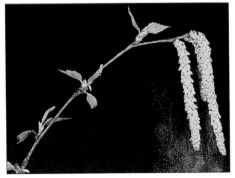

Patients allergic to birch pollen may have cross reactions with some foods (eg, apples, peaches)

Diagnosis

The importance of a careful case history cannot be over-emphasised. The history, supported by diagnostic tests, should point towards a few possible offending foods or groups of foods. A diagnostic diet period is helpful. Usually, a highly restricted diet is not necessary—elimination diets based on essential amino acids are expensive and unpalatable, resulting in low compliance. A diet period of two weeks is usually sufficient, but a more prolonged period may be necessary, especially in the case of atopic dermatitis. To ensure that patients get sufficient nutrition while excluding suspected foods from their diet, the help of a clinical dietitian with experience of food allergy should be enlisted.

Occupational food allergy

Type of reaction	Characteristics	Prevalence
Bakers' asthma (IgE mediated)	Asthma and rhinitis by inhalation of flour	20% of bakers become sensitised during working period of 20 years
Contact urticaria (immunological)	Contact urticaria in persons handling foods (eg, cooks)	Unknown
Contact dermatitis	Contact eczema in persons handling foods (eg, cooks)	Unknown

ABC of Allergies

Testing

Standardised food extracts are rarely available for use in skin prick testing to diagnose food allergy. However, a few food extracts have been validated in clinical trials in children and adults by using a double blind, placebo controlled food challenge as the gold standard. Foods that have been validated in this way include cod, peanuts, cows' milk, hens' eggs, shrimps, and soy beans. In many cases it is better and more convenient to use fresh fruits for skin prick testing. A drop of liquid food or a piece of solid food is placed on the forearm and pricked through (the "prick-prick" method).

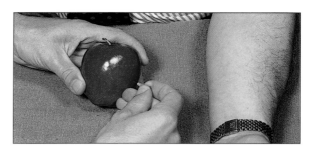
Fresh fruit can be used for skin prick testing for fruit allergy

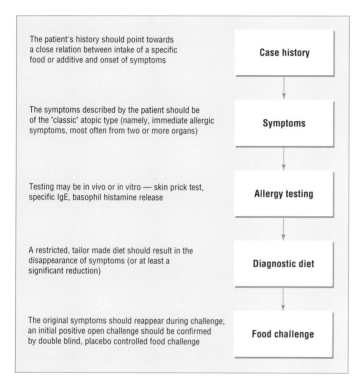

The patient's history should point towards a close relation between intake of a specific food or additive and onset of symptoms	**Case history**
The symptoms described by the patient should be of the "classic" atopic type (namely, immediate allergic symptoms, most often from two or more organs)	**Symptoms**
Testing may be in vivo or in vitro — skin prick test, specific IgE, basophil histamine release	**Allergy testing**
A restricted, tailor made diet should result in the disappearance of symptoms (or at least a significant reduction)	**Diagnostic diet**
The original symptoms should reappear during challenge; an initial positive open challenge should be confirmed by double blind, placebo controlled food challenge	**Food challenge**

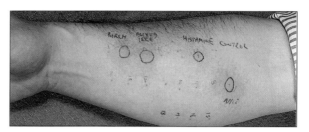
Cross reactivity between birch pollen and apple in patient with springtime hay fever and oral allergy syndrome after ingestion of apple

> **Results of allergen-specific IgE should be interpreted with caustion, especially weakly positive results in patients with high serum concentrations of total IgE**

The same reservations expressed for skin prick testing—namely, poorly standardised food allergen extracts—are also true for the various methods for determining serum concentrations of allergen-specific IgE against food. Another major problem with the newer and technically highly sensitive methods is that they detect the many clinically insignificant serological cross reactions, in which IgE raised against and directed towards epitopes on, for example, grass pollen, also binds to wheat proteins, but without any clinical significance of the finding

The significance of reactions to patch testing is currently being evaluated in several centres. However, before any new test is included for routine diagnosis, it should be validated in clinical trials with a double blind, placebo controlled food challenge as the gold standard.

Confirmation with oral food challenge

Double blind, placebo controlled food challenge may be needed to confirm the medical history of and positive diagnostic tests for food allergy. Most published studies show that in an average of 50% of patients whose medical history plus positive skin prick test result or positive IgE result suggest food allergy, allergy can be confirmed by a double blind, placebo controlled food challenge. Using fresh foods masked in a vehicle is better than using freeze dried foods in capsules. In selected cases an open challenge (that is, not double blind or

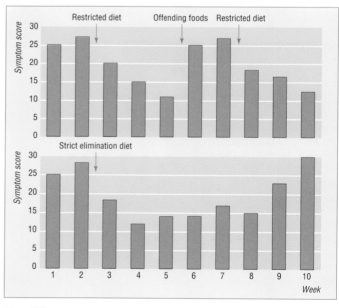
Top: Effect on symptoms of introducing restricted diet (elimination of suspected offending food) then reintroducing normal diet then returning to restricted diet in a patient who was eventually confirmed as being allergic to wheat and rye in a double blind, placebo controlled food challenge. Bottom: Effect on symptoms of a very strict elimination diet in a patient with atopic dermatitis. Although symptoms decreased initially, they had returned to normal levels by week 10 (although the diet was still being maintained). If at week 8 the patient had been given an open challenge or had returned to a normal diet, a food related exacerbation would have been suspected and false conclusions drawn. Especially in diseases with a high degree of spontaneous fluctuations in severity of symptoms a double blind, placebo controlled food challenge is mandatory, and care must be taken to avoid overinterpretation of the results

placebo controlled) may be used; if the results are negative then the patient is not allergic to the offending food, whereas a positive result should be confirmed by a further, double blind, placebo controlled food challenge. Food challenges should be conducted only by staff with specialist training and in the presence of a physician (or a paediatrician, for children aged under 16). They should be conducted cautiously, with incremental doses and with the immediate availability of adrenaline (epinephrine) and other resuscitative measures in view of the small risk of a serious allergic reaction.

Treatment

The only treatment for food allergy is avoidance of the offending food. Training patients to avoid a particular food often requires the help of a dietitian, clear written instructions, and advice about the labelling of foods. Many patients outgrow their clinical reactivity to a food (90% of infants allergic to milk do so by the age of 3, and half of patients who are allergic to eggs do so, but most patients allergic to peanuts or cod do not). The diagnosis should therefore be re-evaluated yearly.

Adrenaline is life saving in cases of anaphylaxis and should be administered as early as possible. It is administered with a user friendly device (see later chapter on anaphylaxis), with careful instruction of patients and, in the case of children, their parents, schoolteachers, etc. Other antiallergy drugs, including cromoglycate and glucocorticoids, have been investigated in clinical trials with conflicting results and are generally unhelpful. Their use should be restricted to selected cases only, with specialist advice. Antihistamines are effective in relieving the symptoms of the oral allergy syndrome but may mask initial warning symptoms of a more severe reaction and should therefore not be used.

Food aversion

Symptoms that cannot be confirmed by double blind, placebo controlled food challenge may none the less be very distressing for patients and are likely to reflect a heterogeneous and largely unexplained group of disorders that include food aversion ("food fads"). Such patients may present with atypical and non-specific symptoms. Although they consider their symptoms to be food induced, they are often unable to identify specific foods or they report foods that are not typical for inducing IgE mediated allergy. Early specialist referral and exclusion of an IgE dependent mechanism (and potential for serious reactions) may be reassuring for the patient and their general practitioner.

The possible role of food allergy in other diseases or behavioural disorders is difficult to establish, although association is often easy to exclude on the basis of the history and the results of diagnostic tests. It is unhelpful to dismiss out of hand the possibility that a patient's symptoms are provoked by food. Equally it is inappropriate to interpret a clinical presentation as food allergy in the absence of any indication of an immunological disorder.

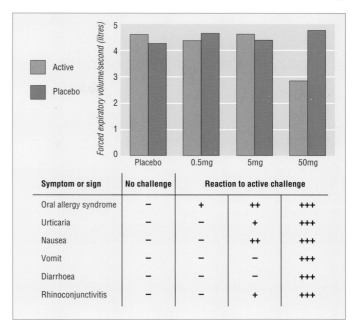

Symptom or sign	No challenge	Reaction to active challenge		
Oral allergy syndrome	−	+	++	+++
Urticaria	−	−	+	+++
Nausea	−	−	++	+++
Vomit	−	−	−	+++
Diarrhoea	−	−	−	+++
Rhinoconjunctivitis	−	−	+	+++

Reaction pattern during titrated double blind, placebo controlled food challenge in patient allergic to eggs. With maximum challenge (50 mg of egg), the patient reacted with a systemic reaction within two minutes of challenge. Blood pressure was maintained. The next day, exacerbation of the patient's atopic dermatitis occurred

> **Prophylaxis with breast feeding or with documented, hypoallergenic hydrolysates is effective against development of allergy to cows' milk and of atopic dermatitis but will not prevent later development of inhalant allergies**

Diseases without proved association to food intake
- Multiple chemical sensitivities
- Chronic fatigue syndrome
- Rheumatoid arthritis
- Hyperactivity disorders
- Depression
- Crohn's disease
- Serous otitis media

Further reading
- Bruinjzeel-Koomen CAFM, Ortolani C, Aas K, Bindslev-Jensen C, Bjorksten B, Moneret Vautrin DA, et al. Position paper. Adverse reactions to foods. *Allergy* 1995;50:623-36
- Høst A. Cow's milk protein allergy and intolerance in infancy. Some clinical, epidemiological and immunological aspects. *Pediatr Allergy Immunol* 1994;5(suppl):5-36
- Lahti A. Non-immunological contact urticaria. *Arch Dermatol* 1980;60(suppl 91):1-49
- Bindslev-Jensen C, Poulsen LK. In vitro diagnostic methods in the diagnosis of food hypersensitivity. In: Metcalfe DD, Sampson H, Simon RA, eds. *Food allergy: adverse reactions to foods and food additives.* 2nd ed. Oxford: Blackwell Science, 1996:137-50

14 Adverse reactions to drugs

Daniel Vervloet, Stephen Durham

Definition

An adverse reaction to a drug has been defined as any noxious or unintended reaction to a drug that is administered in standard doses by the proper route for the purpose of prophylaxis, diagnosis, or treatment. Some drug reactions may occur in everyone, whereas others occur only in susceptible patients. A drug allergy is an immunologically mediated reaction that exhibits specificity and recurrence on re-exposure to the offending drug.

Incidence

Adverse reactions to drugs are very common in everyday medical practice. A French study of 2067 adults aged 20-67 years attending a health centre for a check up reported that 14.7% gave reliable histories of systemic adverse reactions to one or more drugs. In a Swiss study of 5568 hospital inpatients, 17% had adverse reactions to drugs. Fatal drug reactions occur in 0.1% medical inpatients and 0.01% of surgical inpatients. The main drugs implicated are antibiotics and non-steroidal anti-inflammatory drugs. Adverse reactions to drugs occurring during anaesthesia (muscle relaxants, general anaesthetics, and opiates), although less common (1 in 6000 patients receiving anaesthesia), are life threatening, with a mortality of about 6%.

Numerous mechanisms have been implicated in adverse reactions to drugs. However, these mechanisms are not fully understood, which may explain the difficulty in differentiating drug allergy from other forms of drug reactions and in assessing the incidence of drug allergy, evaluating risk factors, and defining management strategies.

Mechanisms

Allergic reactions to drugs are classified according to Coombs' types I-IV. Most drugs (penicillins, sulphonamides) have low molecular weight (haptens) and are bound to proteins before being recognised by lymphocytes or antibodies. Pseudoallergic reactions to drugs may mimic these immunological mechanisms—for example, by direct release of histamine by opioids or complement activation by radioactive contrast media.

Risk factors

Adverse drug reactions occur mainly in young and middle aged adults and are twice as common in women. Genetic factors may be important. A familial predisposition to antimicrobial drugs has recently been reported. The HLA type may predispose to reactions to aspirin (HLA-DQw2) and insulin allergy (B7DR2, DR3). The slow N-acetylation phenotype may predispose to sulphonamide reactions—particularly common in patients with HIV infection. The role of atopy in predisposing to drug reactions is controversial. It may be important in reactions to iodinated contrast material but not to penicillin or reactions during anaesthesia. Risk factors relating to drugs themselves include macromolecular size (large molecules may be complete antigens—for example, insulin); bivalence (ability to cross link receptors—for example, succinyl choline); and the ability to act

---

Classification of adverse reactions to drugs

Reactions that may occur in anyone

Drug overdose—Toxic reactions linked to excess dose or impaired excretion, or to both

Drug side effect—Undesirable pharmacological effect at recommended doses

Drug interaction—Action of a drug on the effectiveness or toxicity of another drug

Reactions that occur only in susceptible subjects

Drug intolerance—A low threshold to the normal pharmacological action of a drug

Drug idiosyncrasy—A genetically determined, qualitatively abnormal reaction to a drug related to a metabolic or enzyme deficiency

Drug allergy—An immunologically mediated reaction, characterised by specificity, transferability by antibodies or lymphocytes, and recurrence on re-exposure

Pseudoallergic reaction—A reaction with the same clinical manifestations as an allergic reaction (eg, as a result of histamine release) but lacking immunological specificity

---

Mechanisms of drug allergy

Type I*	Immediate hypersensitivity, IgE mediated	Anaphylaxis, urticaria, angio-oedema, bronchospasm
Type II	Cytotoxic reactions, IgG and IgM mediated	Cytopenia, vasculitis
Type III	Immune complex reactions, IgG and IgM mediated	Serum sickness, vasculitis
Type IV	Lymphocyte mediated reactions	Contact sensitivity

*Non-specific complement activation and non-specific histamine release may mimic type I reactions

---

Risk factors for drug allergy

Patient related
Age, sex, genetics, atopy, AIDS

Drug related
Macromolecular size; bivalency, haptens; route, dose, duration of treatment

Aggravating factors
β Blockers, asthma, pregnancy

as happens. Sensitisation may be dependent on route of administration; it occurs most commonly with the local route, less commonly with the parenteral route, and least often with the oral route. Intravenous administration gives rise to more severe reactions. β Blocking drugs inhibit the patient's response to adrenaline given to treat anaphylaxis.

> **Asthma and pregnancy may excerbate adverse reactions to drugs**

Diagnosis

Clinical history

Evaluation of drug allergy must begin with a precise and detailed history, including clinical symptoms and their timing and duration in relation to drug exposure. Reactions may be immediate (as in anaphylaxis, bronchospasm, urticaria, or angio-oedema); accelerated (occurring within 3 days (as in urticaria, asthma)); or late (occurring >3 days after first receiving the drug). Late reactions include mucocutaneous syndromes (rashes, exfoliative dermatitis) or haematological type (anaemia, thrombocytopenia, neutropenia).

> **As with other allergic diseases, true drug allergy requires prior exposure (sensitisation), and symptoms occur typically after ther first dose of a subsequent course**

Clinical manifestations of drug allergy

Manifestation	Clinical features	Examples of drugs
Anaphylaxis	Urticaria or angio-oedema, rhinitis, asthma, abdominal pain, cardiovascular collapse	Penicillin, neuromuscular blocking drugs
Pulmonary	Interstitial pneumonitis	Amiodarone, nitrofurantoin chemotherapeutic agents
	Asthma	Aspirin, non-steroidal anti-inflammatory drugs, β blockers
Hepatic	Acute or chronic hepatitis	Halothane, chlorpromazine, carbamazepine
Haematological	Haemolytic anaemia	Penicillin, α-methyldopa, mephenamic acid
	Thrombocytopenia	Frusemide, thiazides, gold salts
	Neutropenia	Penicillin
	Agranulocytosis	Phenylbutazone, chloramphenicol
	Aplastic anaemia	Non-steroidal anti-inflammatory drugs, sulphonamides
Renal	Interstitial nephritis, nephrotic syndrome	Cimetidine
Cardiac	Eosinophilic myocarditis	α-methyldopa
Other	Serum sickness, drug fever, vasculitis, lymphadenopathy	Anticonvulsants, diuretics, antibiotics, hydralazine, procainamide, penicillamine

Diagnostic tests

Skin prick tests may be helpful for diagnosing IgE dependent drug reactions, although occasionally positive results to skin prick testing may result from non-specific histamine release independent of IgE (for example, propofol, atracurium). Radioimmunoassays (for example, the radioallergosorbent test (RAST)) may detect serum IgE antibodies to certain drugs (penicillin and succinyl choline) and latex, which may be responsible for reactions during general anaesthesia that are unrelated to drugs. The same reservations apply as for skin tests.

Tryptase is a valuable marker of mast cell degranulation and may be helpful in the differential diagnosis of anaphylaxis. Serum tryptase concentrations peak one hour after anaphylactic reactions but may be detected several hours later. Serum samples at between 30 minutes and 5 hours after the event, when compared with baseline concentrations taken weeks after, may confirm or exclude the diagnosis.

Immediate skin testing for diagnosing IgE dependent allergy

Antibiotics
- Penicillin
- Cephalosporins

Anaesthetic drugs
- Muscle relaxants
- Thiopentone

Enzymes
- Chymopapain
- Streptokinase

Chemotherapeutic drugs
- Cisplatin

Others
- Insulin, latex

False positive and false negative reactions may occur with these skin tests

Provocation tests

Oral provocation tests, although seldom required, may be regarded as the "gold standard." They must be performed under strict medical supervision with resuscitative equipment available.

Drug reactions and the skin

Drug induced rashes are the commonest side effect of many drugs. In general, the mechanisms are unknown, and only about 10% of such reactions result from true allergic mechanisms. Typical examples of drug induced rashes include erythematous maculopapular eruptions, fixed drug eruptions, erythema multiforme, and exfoliative dermatitis.

Cutaneous reactions to drugs

Manifestation	Examples
Pruritis, urticaria or angio-oedema, maculopapular rash	Most drugs
Contact dermatitis	Antibiotics, ethylenediamine
Photodermatitis	Griseofulvin, sulphonamides
Fixed drug eruption	Metronidazole, penicillin
Toxic epidermal necrosis (potentially life threatening)	Sulphonamides, phenytoin, carbamazepine, barbiturates, allopurinol, etc

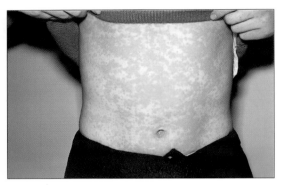

Erythematous maculopapular eruption due to penicillin: rashes of this kind are by far the most common reactions to drugs

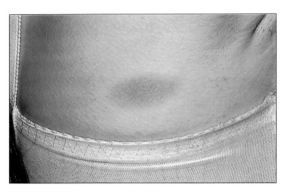

Fixed drug eruption, so called because the lesion recurs at the same site after each administration—in this case, due to barbiturates

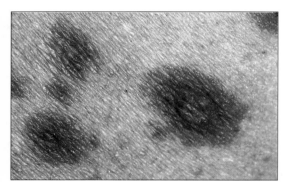

Erythema multiforme due to sulphonamide treatment, showing characteristic target-like lesions

Management

Avoidance

As a general rule, a drug responsible for an allergic reaction should not be reused, unless there is an absolute need and no alternative drug is available. This is seldom the case with antibiotics, the commonest cause of allergic reactions.

Premedication

Pretreatment with H_1 antihistamines should not be used as they do not prevent anaphylactic shock and may mask early signs. However, in association with H_1 antihistamines, corticosteroids have been shown to be effective in reducing reactions to radioactive contrast media.

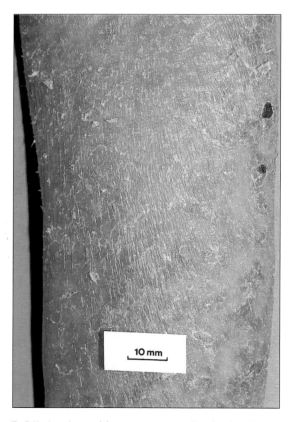

Exfoliative dermatitis—a severe complication in this case due to co-trimoxazole

10 mm

Desensitisation

Desensitisation should be considered in patients who have experienced IgE mediated allergic reactions to penicillin and who require penicillin for the treatment of serious infections—for example, bacterial endocarditis and meningitis. Protocols using oral and parenteral routes have been proposed. Oral administration is preferred because it is less likely to provoke a life threatening reaction. Desensitisation may occasionally be indicated for other antibiotics—for example, sulphonamides, cephalosporins—under specialist supervision.

Diagnosis of specific drug reactions

Muscle relaxants

Muscle relaxants are responsible for an anaphylactic reaction in 1 in 4500 general anaesthesias. The mechanism is IgE dependent. Diagnosis depends on the history supported by a positive result to skin prick testing or presence of serum allergen specific IgE by the radioallergosorbent test, or both of these.

Narcotics

Although opioid analgesics are the most commonly prescribed drugs, anaphylactic reactions are rare. Some narcotics (for example, morphine) are able to induce histamine release. Others, such as fentanyl, do not.

Local anaesthetics

Reactions are seldom related to the local anaesthetic itself. Most general reactions are not allergic but are the result of vasovagal attacks. IgE mediated reactions are the exception. Reactions may be due to adjuvants or preservatives or the injection technique. Associated drugs that may be responsible include adrenaline (epinephrine), sulphites, parabens, antibiotics. Skin prick tests using local anaesthetics are useful although occasional false negative and false positive reactions may occur. They may be used as part of an incremental drug challenge ending with the standard therapeutic dose administered subcutaneously.

Antibiotics

While immediate type reactions to penicillin *may* be diagnosed by skin tests which include both the major determinant (penicilloyl polylysine) and the minor determinant mixture (benzylpenicillin penilloate, MDM), this test is of low specificity and about 50% of patients with a positive reaction have no reaction to subsequent challenge. Skin tests are not helpful for other manifestations of penicillin allergy (contact dermatitis, exfoliative dermatitis, etc). Skin prick tests with other antibiotics (for example, cephalosporins, amoxycillin, clavulinic acid, and aztreonam) may be performed. Skin prick tests with antibiotics other than penicillin have a high false negative rate, although a positive result may provide supportive evidence for a clinical history suggestive of an IgE mediated reaction.

The slides for the four photographs of drug induced skin reactions were provided by Dr Rino Cerio, consultant dermatologist at the Royal London Hospital, and Dr William F Jackson, and published with permission from *A Colour Atlas of Allergic Skin Disorders* (Wolfe, 1992).

Radiocontrast media

- The incidence of reactions to radiocontrast media is between 4.6% and 8.5% of procedures
- Anaphylaxis occurs in 1% and death in 0.001-0.009% of patients who receive radiocontrast media
- The mechanism is unknown but may relate to complement activation
- Newer contrast media with low osmolarity are much safer, although life threatening reactions may still occur
- There are no diagnostic tests
- Atopy is a predisposing factor, and patients with a previous reaction have a 17-35% chance of recurrence on re-exposure
- Prevention of reactions involves the use of newer radiocontrast media and premedication with oral corticosteroids and antihistamines in patients at risk

Aspirin and non-steroidal anti-inflammatory drugs

- Aspirin may induce anaphylaxis, urticaria, asthma, rhinitis, angio-oedema, Lyell's syndrome, purpura, and photodermatitis
- About 20% of asthmatic adults are sensitive to aspirin
- Associated reactions to other non-steroidal anti-inflammatory drugs are common, such that all should be avoided in patients sensitive to aspirin
- The mechanism may be related to inhibition of prostaglandin synthesis with overproduction of leukotrienes
- In cases of diagnostic doubt oral challenges may be performed (these are dangerous in patients with asthma, in whom bronchial inhalation provocation with lysine aspirin is the safer option)
- Paracetamol is tolerated by most but not all patients who are sensitive to non-steroidal anti-inflammatory drugs

> In the rare cases when penicillin desensitisation is indicated, the penicillin is best administered orally in specialist centres—side effects are then infrequent and usually mild (pruritis or rashes)

Further reading

- Pradal M, Vervloet D. Drug reactions. In: Kay AB, ed. *Allergy and allergic diseases.* Oxford: Blackwell Science, 1997:1671-92
- Vervloet D, Pradal M. *Drug allergy.* Sundbyberg: S-M Ewert, 1992
- Sullivan TG. Drug allergy. In: Middleton E, ed. *Allergy: principles and practice.* 4th ed. St Louis, MO: Mosby, 1993:1726-46
- Cerio R, Jackson WF. *A colour atlas of allergic skin disorders.* London: Wolfe, 1992

15 Venom allergy

Pamela W Ewan

Stings from bees and wasps, the most common stinging insects in Britain, can cause severe allergic reactions, including anaphylaxis. Coroners' data suggest that an average of four deaths from bee or wasp stings occur each year in the United Kingdom, but this is almost certainly an underestimate because venom anaphylaxis is not always recognised as the cause of death.

Hymenoptera insects

Classification
The hymenoptera are subdivided into families, including the Apidae (honey bees and bumble bees) and the Vespidae (wasps, hornets, and paper wasps). In Britain most reactions are caused by stings from wasps (the Vespula species) rather than from bees. Reactions to bee stings are almost always associated with the honey bee.

Venoms
Bee and wasp venoms are different, each containing distinct major allergens, which are well defined. Phospholipase A2 and mellitin occur only in bee venom, and antigen 5 only in wasp venom, but both venoms contain hyaluronidases. Patients allergic to wasp venom are rarely allergic to bee venom.

Sensitisation

Most people, unless they have a specific occupational risk, are rarely stung by wasps, perhaps once every 10-15 years. Sensitisation to wasp venom requires only a few stings, and can occur after a single sting.

In contrast, allergy to bee venom occurs mainly in people who have been stung frequently by bees. Thus almost all patients who are allergic to bees are beekeepers or their families, or sometimes their neighbours.

Clinical features

The normal effect of a bee or wasp sting is to cause intense local pain, some immediate erythema, and often a small area (up to 1 cm diameter) of oedema. Allergic reactions can be either local or generalised.

Local reactions
Local reactions involve oedema at the site of the sting. This comes on over several hours and varies in size, but it can affect a hand or even an entire limb. In a dependent area this can lead to blistering and sometimes secondary infection. Such oedema is not dangerous unless it affects the airway.

Generalised reactions
Generalised (or systemic) reactions vary greatly in severity. Early features are erythema and pruritus, followed by urticaria and facial or generalised angio-oedema. Patients with more severe generalised reactions often feel extremely ill, as if they are going to die ("a sense of impending doom"). Dyspnoea often occurs and can be due either to laryngeal oedema or to

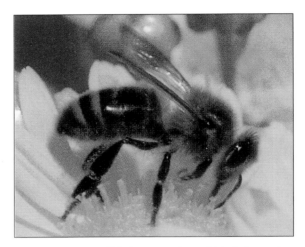
Honet bee (*Apis mellifera*): 1.5 cm long, fairly hairy and brown with abdominal bands

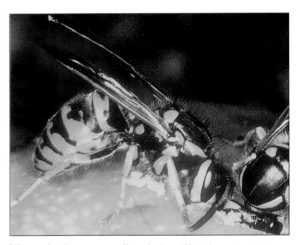
Wasp, also known as yellow jacket (*Vespula* spp) ≤ 1.5 cm long; yrllow and black striped abdomen; typical waist; and little hair

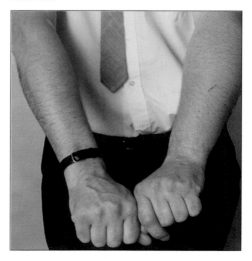
Patient with angio-oedema of the left forearm: local allergic reaction to a bee sting

asthma. In severe reactions hypotension occurs, causing lightheadedness, giddiness, fainting, or loss of consciousness. Other less common features are abdominal pain, incontinence, central chest pain, or visual disturbances.

The clinical picture is variable—patients may have only erythema, urticaria, and angio-oedema or may develop loss of consciousness, with few warning symptoms, within minutes of a sting. The onset of generalised reactions is early, usually within 10 minutes of a sting.

Diagnosis

Venom allergy is diagnosed from the history of the allergic reaction, backed up by tests for venom-specific IgE antibodies. It is important to check the basis of the patient's assertion about the type of insect responsible for the sting. Many patients say the sting is from a bee when it is in fact a wasp sting. The vast majority of patients (except beekeepers etc) will be wasp allergic. Accurate diagnosis is important as it has implications for management.

The history should be confirmed by demonstrating, by skin test or blood test, specific IgE; this is essential if desensitisation is considered as a treatment. Skin tests—either skin prick tests or intradermal tests with bee and wasp venom and the appropriate positive and negative controls—are more accurate but should be done by allergists as skin tests for venom are more difficult to interpret than skin tests for inhaled allergens. Alternatively, serum bee-specific and wasp-specific IgE can be measured by a radioallergosorbent test (RAST), CAP-RAST, or other assays.

It is important to be aware that since the introduction of the more sensitive CAP-RAST, there have been more (up to 30%) false positive results—that is, patients with serum IgE to both bee and wasp venom (double positives) when they are allergic to only one venom. However, double positives can occur even with the radioallergosorbent test (in about 6% of cases). The term allergy refers to a state of clinical reactivity and is not the same as sensitisation (presence of specific IgE antibodies), which can occur without clinical reactivity. Patients are rarely allergic to both bee and wasp venom. This means that if the history is not checked, and venom IgE to only a single venom is measured, the wrong diagnosis can result. Studies in the general population show that some subjects who have a history of stings but no reactions have venom-specific IgE.

Acute management

Local reactions
Acute management should be with oral antihistamines, which may be required for several days. A quick acting drug should be used (for example, one of the newer, non-sedative antihistamines). Very large swellings may require intramuscular antihistamines and steroids. Prevention is more effective, and the patient should take a large dose of an antihistamine (double the standard dose) immediately after being stung, before the localised reaction is established, to abrogate incipient angio-oedema.

Generalised allergic reactions
Management depends on the severity and the particular features of the reaction, as for any systemic allergic reaction. Cutaneous reactions require oral antihistamines or injected chlorpheniramine. Moderate reactions often require intramuscular chlorpheniramine and hydrocortisone, and treatment for asthma—for example, inhaled $\beta2$ agonists—may be necessary. Severe reactions, including those with marked respiratory difficulty or hypotension, should be treated with

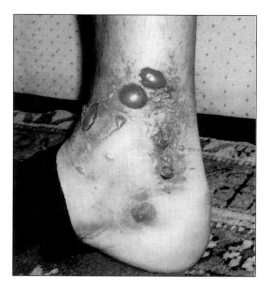

Patient with angio-oedema and blistering of the ankle: local allergic reaction to a bee sting

---

Natural course

- A substantial proportion of patients (20-80% in different studies) with a history of a generalised reaction to a sting have no such reaction to a subsequent sting—that is, spontaneous improvement is common
- Less severe generalised reactions may also occur
- However, the course can be variable—a series of stings may result in a generalised reaction, no reaction, and then another generalised reaction
- Children do particularly well: one study showed that 95% of those with a history of mild generalised reactions had no reaction to a subsequent sting
- The next sting will not necessarily cause a more severe reaction, but patients in accident and emergency departments are often told that it will
- Reasons for the variable outcome are not well understood but include the interval from the last sting (the longer the interval the lower the risk of another generalised reaction), the patient's immune response at the time of the sting (this will change with time), the dose of venom injected, and the site of the sting

---

Drugs used in acute management of reactions to stings

Type of reaction	Treatment
Local*	Antihistamines (oral)
Systemic†:	
Mild	Antihistamines (oral or intramuscular)
Moderate	Antihistamines (intramuscular); hydrocortisone (intramuscular); inhaled $\beta2$ agonist (if asthma); inhaled adrenaline (if laryngeal oedema)
Severe	Adrenaline (intramuscular); chlorpheniramine (intramuscular or slow intravenous); hydrocortisone (intramuscular or slow intravenous)

The distinction between categories of systemic reaction may be blurred. If in doubt, treat as for the most severe category.
*Treatment is usually required for several days.
†Single dose is often sufficient.

adrenaline (intramuscular) followed by chlorpheniramine and hydrocortisone. Other measures, including intravenous fluids, may also be required, but, provided that treatment is started soon after the onset of the reaction, the drugs above are usually all that are needed.

> **Adrenaline (intramuscular) is the key drug for severe reactions**

Further management

After a generalised reaction, patients need further advice and ideally should be referred to an allergy clinic specialising in venom allergy. As there are not many of these in Britain, general practitioners should be aware that there are two options for further management: patients can either be desensitised or be given the appropriate drugs to treat a reaction themselves. To choose the appropriate management, it helps to classify general reactions by severity.

Who should be desensitised?

Desensitisation (immunotherapy)
Among patients with generalised reactions, those with severe reactions usually require desensitisation, those with mild reactions do not, and those with moderate reactions may or may not. Other factors—such as the risk of a future sting, the interval from the last sting, other medical problems, the ability of the patient to treat himself or herself, and access to medical help—may influence the decision.

Before desensitisation is given the nature of the sting must be accurately diagnosed and venom-specific IgE demonstrated.

The indications in Britain for desensitisation are conservative (in some countries any patient with a generalised reaction, no matter how trivial, would be desensitised). This is because, although immunotherapy for hymenoptera venom is highly effective, the high incidence of spontaneous improvement, as well as the side effects of treatment, has to be taken into account. Venom immunotherapy carries a risk (of about 10%) of inducing systemic allergic reactions and can produce anaphylaxis. It should therefore be performed only in specialist centres treating an adequate number of patients each year.

Self medication for future reactions
Those not being desensitised should be given oral antihistamines to take if they are stung again. They should take the antihistamines as soon as they are stung to modify or abort reactions. In a patient with a mild generalised reaction this is normally sufficient. Those with moderate or severe reactions should also be given syringes preloaded with adrenaline. They administer a dose of 0.3mg (0.3ml of 1/1000 strength) intramuscularly for adults and children from age 5 years. A syringe containing a smaller dose (0.15 mg) suitable for younger children is available, but children with venom allergy rarely need this. If other drugs are required these should be given by doctors or paramedics. All patients should seek the assistance of an adult as soon as they are stung, in case medical help is required.

What does immunotherapy involve?
Various regimens are available. Conventional immunotherapy, the standard one, entails an initial course of weekly injections over three months, starting with low doses of venom and reaching the highest dose of $100\mu g$ (equivalent to two stings). Thereafter, maintenance injections of the same dose are given at monthly or longer intervals for three years. The treatment can be given only in specialist centres, where

Classification of systemic allergic reactions to bee or wasp stings

Severity	Symbol	Reactions
Mild	+	Erythema, pruritus, urticaria, angio-oedema, rhinitis, nausea
Moderate	+ +	Mild asthma, angio-oedema, abdominal pain
Severe	+ + +	Respiratory difficulty (laryngeal oedema or asthma), marked hypotension, collapse, loss of consciousness

Indications for venom immunotherapy

Type of reaction	Venom-specific IgE	Venom immunotherapy
Severe systemic (cardiovascular and/or respiratory symptoms)	Positive	Yes
Moderate systemic (angio-oedema, mild asthma, or lightheadedness etc)	Positive	Sometimes, but usually not
Mild systemic (urticaria, angio-oedema)	Positive	No

> **Syringes preloaded with adrenaline (for example, EpiPen or Anapen (which is available on a named patient basis)) are available by using the standard prescription form**

Value of self medication
- The main advantage of self medication is that reactions are treated only if they occur
- This is sensible because most patients (except beekeepers) are not stung again for years, and the next sting may cause no reaction or a less severe one
- The disadvantage is that one cannot be certain that the appropriate drugs (especially adrenaline) will be given (early treatment of anaphylaxis is highly effective)
- The decision on self medication should be reached on an individual basis after balancing all factors and bearing in mind that desensitisation is not without risk

resuscitation facilities exist, to conform with the guidelines of the Committee on the Safety of Medicines (1986 and 1994), because of the risk of side effects. Drugs to treat anaphylaxis must be immediately available, and patients have to be kept under observation for one hour after each injection. Although highly effective, immunotherapy is expensive and time consuming.

Mechanism of immunotherapy

T cells secrete cytokines which orchestrate the immune response. T helper (Th) cells are subdivided into Th1 and Th2 subsets, on the basis of their cytokine secreting profile in response to stimulation with antigen or allergen.

It has been shown that venom immunotherapy leads to marked changes in cytokine secretion patterns, with a switch from the abnormal Th2 cytokine response to a Th1 response. This may be due to downregulation of the Th2 response (anergy) or immune deviation in favour of a Th1 response, or to both these. The Th2 subset of Th cells produces interleukin 4, interleukin 5, and interleukin 3, which are proallergic, leading to IgE synthesis (interleukin 4) and activating or attracting eosinophils (interleukin 5) and mast cells (interleukin 3). Venom immunotherapy leads to loss of secretion of Th2 cytokines in response to venom stimulation, and, instead, Th1 cytokine production (interleukin 2 and interferon gamma) is induced. Interferon gamma opposes the effect of interleukin 4 in inducing B cells to secrete IgE.

This cytokine switch will lead in the long term to loss of IgE synthesis and the allergic response but does not explain the fact that, clinically, desensitisation occurs before these changes take place. This suggests that other, earlier operating mechanisms are involved.

The table on classification of systemic reactions is adapted from *Allergy and Allergic Diseases*, Kay AB, ed (Insect-sting allergy (Ewan PW)): Blackwell Science, 1997.

Immunotherapy is highly effective in selected cases

Can we predict the outcome of a future sting?

- There is no blood test that will reliably predict how a patient will react to a future sting
- No direct correlation exists between the concentration of venom-specific IgG in the serum and protection from the next sting
- There may be no reaction to a sting in spite of the presence of venom IgE
- Venom IgE will eventually disappear, but this can take many years. Once it has disappeared completely—both from the serum and from the mast cells—a sting cannot produce a reaction
- Provocation tests are done either with a real sting or with a subcutaneous injection of pure venom. These are the only tests that will reliably show a patient's reactivity, but, although they are very useful, they are not very practicable. Their use is restricted to specialist centres, and they are useful in research

---

Further reading

- Egner W, Ward C, Brown DL, Ewan PW. The incidence and clinical significance of specific IgE to both wasp (vespula) and bee (apis) venom in the same patient. *Clin Exp Allergy* 1998;28:26-34
- McHugh SM, Deighton J, Stewart AG, Lachmann PJ, Ewan PW. Bee venom immunotherapy induces a shift in cytokine responses from a TH-2 to a TH-1 dominant pattern: comparison of rush and conventional immunotherapy. *Clin Exp Allergy* 1995;25:828-38
- Kampelmacher MJ, van der Zwan JC. Provocation test with a living insect as a diagnostic tool in systemic reactions to bee and wasp venom: a prospective study with emphasis on the clinical aspects. *Clin Allergy* 1987;17:317-27
- Valentine MD, Schuberth KC, Kagey-Sobotka A, Graft DF, Kwiterovich KA, Szkalo M, et al. The value of immunotherapy with venom in children with allergy to insect stings. *N Engl J Med* 1990;323:1601-3
- Kay AB, ed. Position paper on allergen immunotherapy: report of a British Society for Allergy and Clinical Immunology Working Party. *Clin Exp Allergy* 1993;23(suppl 3):19-22

16 Anaphylaxis

Pamela W Ewan

Anaphylaxis and anaphylactic death are becoming more common and particularly affect children and young adults. Anaphylaxis can be frightening to deal with because of its rapid onset and severity. Doctors in many fields, but particularly those working in general practice and in accident and emergency departments, need to know how to treat it.

Definition

Anaphylaxis means a severe systemic allergic reaction. No universally accepted definition exists because anaphylaxis comprises a constellation of features, and the argument arises over which features are essential features. A good working definition is that it involves one of the two severe features: respiratory difficulty (which may be due to laryngeal oedema or asthma) and hypotension (which can present as fainting, collapse, or loss of consciousness). Other features are usually present.

The confusion arises because systemic allergic reactions can be mild, moderate, or severe. For example, generalised urticaria, angio-oedema, and rhinitis would not be described as anaphylaxis, as neither respiratory difficulty nor hypotension—the potentially life threatening features—is present.

Mechanism

An allergic reaction results from the interaction of an allergen with specific IgE antibodies, bound to Fc receptors for IgE on mast cells and basophils. This leads to activation of the mast cell and release of preformed mediators stored in granules (including histamine), as well as of newly formed mediators, which are synthesised rapidly. These mediators are responsible for the clinical features. Rapid systemic release of large quantities of mediators will cause capillary leakage and mucosal oedema, resulting in shock and asphyxia.

Anaphylactoid reactions are caused by activation of mast cells and release of the same mediators, but without the involvement of IgE antibodies. For example, certain drugs act directly on mast cells. For practical purposes (management) it is not necessary to distinguish an anaphylactic from an anaphylactoid reaction. This difference is relevant only when investigations are being considered.

Incidence

Hardly any data exist on the overall incidence of anaphylaxis. One recent study examining cases of anaphylaxis presenting to an accident and emergency department in Cambridge (to which all cases from a defined area would be brought) found that 1 in 1500 patients attending the department had anaphylaxis with loss of consciousness or collapse (equivalent to 1 in 10 000 a year in the population) and that the rate almost trebled when systemic allergic reactions with respiratory difficulty were included. Most other data relate to specific causes—for example, anaphylaxis due to allergy to penicillin or to anaesthetic drugs—and are quite variable.

Features of anaphylaxis

- Erythema
- Pruritus (generalised)
- Urticaria
- Angio-oedema
- Laryngeal oedema
- Asthma
- Rhinitis
- Conjunctivitis
- Itching of palate or external auditory meatus
- Nausea, vomiting, abdominal pain
- Palpitations
- Sense of impending doom
- Fainting, lightheadedness
- Collapse
- Loss of consciousness

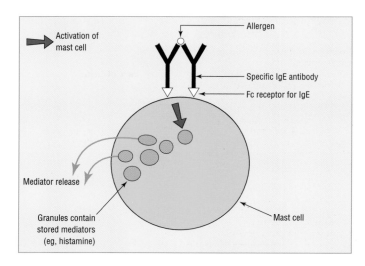

Activation of mast cells by allergen crosslinking of adjacent IgE on cell surface in a type I allergic reaction

Effects of mast cell mediators

Physiological effect	Clinical expression	Danger
Capillary leakage	Urticaria	
	Angio-oedema	
	Laryngeal oedema	Asphyxia
	Hypotension	Shock
Mucosal oedema	Laryngeal oedema	Asphyxia
	Rhinitis	
	Asthma	Respiratory arrest
Smooth muscle contraction	Asthma	Respiratory arrest
	Abdominal pain	

Aetiology

Foods are the commonest cause of anaphylaxis, and evidence suggests that this is an increasing problem, now documented for allergies to peanuts and other nuts. Insect venom is the next most common cause of anaphylaxis. A rapidly increasing problem is allergy to latex rubber. This is probably related to the enormous increase in the use of latex rubber gloves by medical and paramedical staff, as well as to the increase in atopy. Rare causes include exercise, vaccines, and semen. Allergen immunotherapy (desensitisation) may induce anaphylaxis.

Clinical features

It is important to recognise that the picture will vary with the cause. When an allergen is injected systemically (insect stings, intravenous drugs) cardiovascular problems, especially hypotension and shock, predominate. This is especially true when large boluses are given intravenously, as at induction of anaesthesia. Foods that are absorbed transmucosally (from the oral mucosa down) seem especially to cause lip, facial, and laryngeal oedema. Respiratory difficulty therefore predominates. With severe reactions onset occurs soon after exposure (within minutes), and progression is rapid.

Common causes of anaphylaxis

- Foods
- Bee and wasp stings
- Drugs
- Latex rubber

Foods causing anaphylaxis

- Peanuts
- Tree nuts (eg, brazil nut, almond, hazelnut)
- Fish
- Shellfish
- Egg
- Milk
- Sesame
- Pulses (other than peanuts)
- Others

Drugs causing anaphylaxis or anaphylactoid reactions

- Antibiotics (especially penicillin)
- Intravenous anaesthetic drugs
- Aspirin
- Non-steroidal anti-inflammatory drugs
- Intravenous contrast media
- Opioid analgesics

Four brief case histories

Case 1—Woman aged 30, six months pregnant
- Trigger: Chinese meal
- Symptoms and treatment: one hour after start of meal felt faint; mild asthma; severe dyspnoea and laryngeal oedema; loss of consciousness; taken to accident and emergency department after 10 minutes; on arrival cyanosed, respiratory arrest; periorbital oedema; salbutamol infusion; cardiac arrest four minutes later; adrenaline given; intubated with difficulty and ventilated
- Recovered (see figure next page)
- Cause: allergy to green pepper

Case 3—Boy aged 8 months
- Trigger: Tiny quantity of peanut butter
- Symptoms: blisters around mouth; distressed; vomiting; dyspnoea; urticaria
- Cause: allergy to peanuts

Case 2—Woman aged 30
- Trigger: one teaspoonful muesli
- Symptoms and treatment: immediate itching of mouth; throat swollen and uncomfortable inside; vomited; dyspnoea (could not breathe, different from her asthma); laryngeal oedema (obstruction in throat); lightheaded; no loss of consciousness; used her own salbutamol inhaler (no effect); taken to accident and emergency department; respiratory distress; intense erythema and generalised urticaria; given intramuscular adrenaline and chlorpheniramine
- Rapid recovery
- Cause: allergy to brazil nuts and hazelnuts

Case 4—Woman aged 26
- Trigger: vaginal examinations during labour
- Symptoms: itching of vulva; oedema of labia; generalised urticaria and pruritus; mild dyspnoea; felt woozy, lightheaded, odd, shaking
- Cause: allergy to latex rubber

Latex rubber anaphylaxis—unusually—develops more slowly (30 minutes or longer from the time of exposure), as the allergen has to be absorbed through the skin or mucosa (for example, during abdominal or gynaecological surgery, vaginal examination, dental work, or simply contact with, or wearing, rubber gloves). Healthcare workers are especially at risk.

Investigations

The only immediate test that is useful at the time of reaction is mast cell tryptase. Tryptase is released from mast cells in both anaphylactic and anaphylactoid reactions. It is an indicator of mast cell activation but does not distinguish mechanisms or throw light on causes. It is usually but not always raised in severe reactions but may not be in less severe systemic reactions. As mast cell tryptase is only raised transiently, blood should be taken when it peaks at about an hour after the onset of the reaction. This test remains to be fully evaluated.

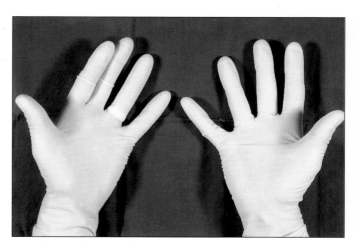

Allergy to latex rubber is common in healthcare workers

Management

Adrenaline (epinephrine) is the most important drug for anaphylaxis and should be given intramuscularly. It is almost always effective.

This should be followed by chlorpheniramine and hydrocortisone (intramuscular or slow intravenous). This is usually all that is required, provided that treatment is started early. Treatment failure is more likely if administration of adrenaline is delayed. Biphasic reactions have been described but are probably rare; administration of hydrocortisone should minimise the risk of late relapse.

Difficulties may arise if the clinical picture is evolving when the patient is first assessed. Adrenaline should be given to all patients with respiratory difficulty or hypotension. If these features are absent but there are other features of a systemic allergic reaction, it is appropriate to give chlorpheniramine and hydrocortisone and reassess. If in doubt, give 500 µg adrenaline intramuscularly in an adult or the appropriate dose in a child.

There can be risks associated with intravenous adrenaline. Adrenaline should not be given intravenously except under special circumstances: profound shock (which is immediately life threatening) or during anaesthesia. Even then, if intravenous adrenaline is given, a dilute solution (1 in 10 000) must be administered very slowly in aliquots (with a maximum initial dose of 100 µg (that is, 1 ml)) with cardiac monitoring. Such treatment therefore is rarely indicated outside hospital.

Although myocardial infarction has been reported in the literature as being associated with the use of adrenaline, this reflects a bias in reporting, as the effective and safe use of adrenaline is not considered worth reporting. Those with wide experience of its use find adrenaline extremely safe.

β Blockers may increase the severity of an anaphylactic reaction and may antagonise some of the beneficial actions of adrenaline. However, if a patient with anaphylaxis is taking β blockers this should not prevent the use of adrenaline.

Supporting treatments

If the patient has hypotension then he or she should lie flat with the legs raised, but if respiratory difficulty is the dominant problem it may be better for the patient to sit up. Oxygen should be administered.

An inhaled $\beta2$ agonist should be given if there is asthma. Inhaled adrenaline is effective for mild to moderate laryngeal oedema but would not be given if intramuscular adrenaline had already been given as first line treatment, and it is not a substitute for intramuscular adrenaline. If drugs are not rapidly effective for shock, intravenous fluids should be given rapidly.

Do not give adrenaline intravenously except in special circumstances (see text)

Drug treatment of anaphylaxis in adults
- *Intramuscular* adrenaline 0.5 ml (500 µg), 1 in 1000 solution (1 mg/ml)
- Intramuscular or slow intravenous chlorpheniramine 10 mg
- Intramuscular or slow intravenous hydrocortisone 200 mg

Doses of intramuscular adrenaline in children

Age (years)	Volume of 1 in 1000 strength (1 mg/ml)	Dose (µg)
1	0.1 ml	100
2-3	0.2 ml*	200
4-7	0.3 ml*	300
8-11	0.4 ml*	400
>11	0.5 ml*	500

This is a guide based on average weight for different age bands. No evidence exists for particular doses for different age bands, and published schedules therefore differ. *Reduce dose in children of below average weight.

Key to management of anaphylaxis
- Awareness
- Recognise it (consider in differential diagnosis)
- Treat quickly
- Deaths in otherwise healthy young people could then be avoided

---

Analphylaxis is easily treatable, and patients can make a complete recovery

---

08.40 Miraculous recovery: Post extubation; stridor responding to nebulised adrenaline. Kept on nebulisation overnight. Patient has full recall of events up to collapsing in restaurant. Alert and responsive apparently no intellectual impairment.

Entry in patient's hospital notes (case 1, box previous page) 9 hours after analphylaxis with cardiorespiratory arrest, showing effectiveness of prompt treatment

Long term management

Patients are commonly sent home from accident and emergency departments without further advice. Patients are not infrequently given an ampoule of adrenaline or a preloaded adrenaline syringe without instruction. This is of little or no value and frightens patients.

It is important to refer patients to an allergist— ideally, one with expertise in anaphylaxis. The cause should be determined, and advice given on avoidance to prevent further attacks. The cause is determined by taking a detailed and structured allergy history, then, in the case of IgE mediated reactions, confirmed (for most allergens) by skin prick tests. The cause is sometimes obvious from the history (as in case 3, previous page, where a typical reaction immediately followed ingestion of peanut butter). In case 1 the cause was also indicated by the history as there had been two allergic reactions, the first milder one after a "ploughman's lunch" with few ingredients and the second after a large Chinese meal containing at least six suspected allergens. Green pepper was the common factor. Skin tests (directly through the flesh of green pepper and also with an aqueous extract of green pepper that we prepared) were strongly positive, confirming the diagnosis.

Early self treatment is highly effective, and reactions can usually be stopped easily. Syringes preloaded with adrenaline are easy for patients to use and readily available. They deliver fixed intramuscular doses and are available in two strengths: for adults (containing 0.3 ml of 1 in 1000 strength (that is, 300 µg)) and for children (0.3 ml of 1 in 2000 (150 µg)). The appropriate self treatment varies and may include other drugs. This should be determined by a specialist as, once a cause is determined and avoidance measures are in place, further reactions after inadvertent exposure are usually less severe. A written treatment plan should be provided by the allergist, and the patient (and relatives) should be taught how and when to use the treatments provided—for example, trainer syringes are available.

To be of help to children, schools and nurseries need training. Some allergists have developed links with community paediatricians, whose teams are best placed to deliver training. This requires expertise, which is now developed in only a few centres. The team in Cambridge is therefore coordinating the production of national guidelines.

If there is no local allergist the general practitioner or the doctor in the accident and emergency department should provide the drugs for self treatment, but it is essential that these are given with advice and training. Practice nurses should have trainer syringes for this purpose.

What to do after an anaphylactic reaction

Action	Aim
Take blood at 1-2 hours for measurement of mast cell tryptase	To confirm anaphylaxis or anaphylactoid reaction
Refer to an allergy clinic to determine cause	To prevent further attacks
Organise self treatment of future reactions (best done by an allergist)	To prevent morbidity (early treatment is the key)

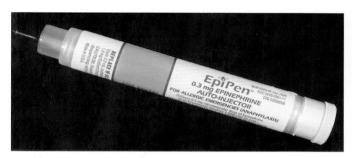

Preloaded adrenaline syringes are available for self treatment of anaphylaxis

> **Some patients who have had an anaphylactic reaction wear a Medic Alert bracelet or necklace—with an inscription endorsed by a doctors that alerts other doctors to the possible cause of any future reaction**

Further reading

- Stewart AG, Ewan PW. The incidence, aetiology and management of anaphylaxis presenting to an accident and emergency department. *Q J Med* 1996;89:859-64
- Fisher MMcD, Baldo BA. The incidence and clinical features of anaphylactic reactions during anaesthesia in Australia. *Ann Fr Anesth Reanim* 1993;12:97-104
- Ewan PW. Clinical study of peanut and nut allergy in 62 consecutive patients: new features and associations. *BMJ* 1996;312:1074-8
- Turjanmaa K, Alenius H, Makinen-Kiljunen S, Reunala T, Palosuo T. Natural rubber latex allergy. *Allergy* 1996;51:593-602
- Vickers DW, Maynard L, Ewan PW. Management of children with potential anaphylactic reactions in the community: a training package and proposal for good practice. *Clin Exp Allergy* 1997;27:898-903

17 Allergy in general practice

Sue Cross, Sallie Buck, Jane Hubbard

In parallel with the known increases in atopy (confirmed by a positive response in skin prick testing to one or more common allergens) and allergy there has been a marked increase in the proportion of general practitioner consultations for asthma, hay fever, and eczema. A greater awareness of the importance of allergy should lead to better diagnosis and management of allergy. This is essential for perennial allergic asthma in children and adults, in whom environmental control and allergen avoidance measures directed against house dust mites are of proved value in reducing asthma symptoms and bronchial hyperresponsiveness. It seems likely that these factors also reduce the need for drug treatment.

Rhinitis symptoms commonly have an allergic aetiology and may be seasonal or perennial. They may be responsible for severe impairment of quality of life. Rhinitis symptoms are frequently trivialised and misdiagnosed by both patients and doctors as "the permanent cold." This is unfortunate as avoidance measures combined with either topical corticosteroids or antihistamines, or both, are extremely effective in controlling symptoms with minimal side effects. Recent surveys have suggested that up to 80% of people with asthma also have rhinitis; treating rhinitis in such people has been shown to reduce asthma symptoms and bronchial hyperresponsiveness.

Role of the practice nurse

The practice nurse has a major (and now established) role in the routine care of asthmatic patients in general practice. It seems logical that this role of the specially trained nurse could be extended, with the support of the general practitioner, to include the recognition and treatment of the allergic component of asthma and also rhinitis.

The extent of the nurse's role depends on many factors, including skills, training, and knowledge. The knowledge base and skills of the doctor and the circumstances of the practice will similarly have an impact. Inquiry about allergic triggers in asthma should be routine in any asthma clinic.

An important question is whether this role should be extended to include more detailed inquiry and use of a simple range of skin prick tests. This issue is particularly important in Britain, which, in contrast to Europe and the United States, has few specialist allergy clinics in the NHS. By spending dedicated time with patients, or by enabling the doctor to spend more time with them, the trained nurse has an immense contribution to make to the task of improving management of asthma and allergy.

Allergy diagnosis in general practice

Accurate allergy diagnosis may be limited by the availability of consultation time. None the less, time taken early on in obtaining a full history may well save time later. Patients should be allowed to explain their symptoms in their own time. At the end of the consultation it is often helpful to ask the patient, "what is your main problem?"

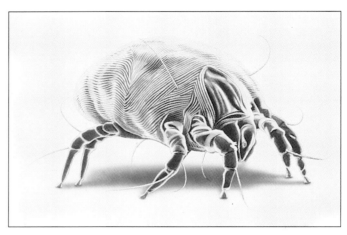

House dust mite, the major cause of perennial allergy in Britain

---

Some common problems (such as adverse reactions to drugs) and less common conditions (such as occupational asthma and anaphylaxis) that are due to allergy may be life threatening and require referral to a specialist allergy clinic

---

Allergic problems in general practice
- Asthma
- Rhinitis—both seasonal (hay fever) and perennial
- Conjunctivitis
- Eczema, particularly in young children
- Occupational asthma
- Food intolerance
- Anaphylaxis—most often provoked by stinging insects, foods such as peanuts and shellfish, or drugs

---

Allergy history in general practice
- Symptoms: past and present; frequency and severity; seasonal or perennial; provoking factors
- Impact on lifestyle: absence from work or school; leisure time; sleep
- Nature of occupation and hobbies
- Treatment: past and present; compliance; efficacy; side effects
- Allergens in the home
- Asthma, eczema, rhinitis, or drug or food allergy: past and present
- Family history of allergic disease
- Main problem?

Skin prick tests

Skin prick testing identifies IgE sensitivity to common allergens, allows diagnosis (or exclusion) of atopy, and provides helpful objective information that should be interpreted in the context of the clinical history of symptoms (or lack of symptoms) on exposure to relevant allergens in the indoor and outdoor environment or workplace. Although skin prick testing with aeroallergens is a simple and safe procedure, it requires training in technique and, more important, in interpretation of the results. Measurement of serum allergen specific IgE, an alternative to skin tests, is done in most district hospitals.

Whether skin prick testing should be performed routinely in general practice in Britain remains a matter of debate. A pilot study evaluated skin prick testing in children and adults in 320 patients in 16 general practices in Britain. The study involved two days' training in allergy, combined with instruction in skin prick testing with four common allergens (and positive and negative controls). The participating nurses found that the techniques were simple, relatively easy to incorporate into their routine assessment of new referrals to the asthma clinic, and acceptable to both adults and children. The nurses also found the techniques acceptable. The procedure undoubtedly increased the nurses' awareness of the role of allergy in patients' asthma, although further studies should look at specific outcome measures. An important finding was the value of negative results of skin prick tests, which excluded atopy in these patients and enabled the investigators to advise patients against inappropriate allergen avoidance measures. A further important advantage was the visual illustration provided by positive results of skin tests, which could be used to reinforce the need for allergen avoidance.

Important practical considerations include the avoidance of use of antihistamines before skin prick testing. In general, when there is concordance between the clinical history and skin prick testing, management is straightforward. For example, an asthmatic patient who has symptoms on exposure to cats or dust and in whom there is an objective confirmation (from skin prick testing) should receive appropriate advice on avoidance. Similarly, a negative history together with negative results of skin prick testing excludes the need for allergen avoidance. When results are discordant (positive history with negative results, or vice versa) they may indicate the need for referral to a specialist. Skin prick tests with common aeroallergens are safe and may be performed by the practice nurse. However, in view of the theoretical risk (albeit remote) associated with giving allergens, injectable adrenaline should be available. Skin prick testing in general practice may be restricted to the four common allergens (house dust mite, cat, dog, grass) and controls (histamine and allergen diluent). Patch testing for suspected contact allergy is complex and should be performed by a specialist dermatologist.

Management of allergy in general practice

If an allergen has been identified as contributing to or causing disease then consideration should be given to the need for measures for avoiding that allergen. These measures should be regarded as complementary to drug treatment. This should not detract from time given to advising patients on the need to take prophylactic drugs regularly—for example, regular inhaled corticosteroids for asthma. In practice, total avoidance, especially of aeroallergens, may be very difficult, so the aim is to reduce overall exposure as much as possible.

Skin prick testing: practice points
- Always check that the patient is not taking antihistamines before performing skin prick tests
- Always include positive (histamine) and negative (allergen diluent) control tests
- In a positive result the weal is (arbitrarily) $\geqslant 2$mm greater than that for the negative control
- Skin prick tests should be performed on the flexor aspect of the forearm with a sterile lancet. The procedure should not be painful or draw blood
- Oral corticosteroids do not significantly inhibit allergen skin prick tests
- Dermatographism may confound results (although it is evident as a positive response at the negative control site)
- Skin prick tests should not be performed if the patient has severe eczema
- Measurement of allergen specific IgE concentrations (radio-allergosorbent test (RAST)) is an alternative if skin prick tests cannot be performed

Advising patients on basis of history and skin prick tests

Allergy history	Skin prick test	Advice
Positive	Positive	Allergen avoidance where appropriate*
Negative	Negative	No need for allergen avoidance
Positive	Negative	Referral to an NHS allergist or an organ based physician with an interest in allergy
Negative	Positive	Referral to an NHS allergist or an organ based physician with an interest in allergy

*In cases of severe hay fever and venom anaphylaxis, refer to specialist for consideration for allergen injection immunotherapy.

Companies supplying skin prick testing kits
- Allerayde, 3 Sanigar Court, Whittle Close, Newark, Nottinghamshire NG24 2BW (tel: 01636 613444)
- ALK Abello (UK), 8 Bennet Road, Reading, Berkshire RG2 0QX (tel: 0118 931 3200)
- Diagenics, 3 Sanigar Court, Whittle Close, Newark, Nottinghamshire NG24 2BW (tel: 01636 605150)

> **For anaphylaxis total avoidance of the relevant allergen is necessary**

ABC of Allergies

Summary of approach for treating common allergic disorders

Rhinitis	Conjunctivitis	Asthma	Eczema	Food allergy/anaphylaxis
Allergen avoidance	Allergen avoidance	Allergen avoidance	Allergen avoidance	Allergen avoidance (may be life saving)
Antihistamine tablets or nasal spray	Antihistamine tablets	Bronchodilator inhaler as required	Soap substitute and regular use of emollients	Specialist referral (for *all* cases of anaphylaxis) and need for dietetic support
Corticosteroid nasal spray (cromoglycate first line in children)	Cromoglycate or nedocromil eye drops	Corticosteroid inhaler (cromoglycate or nedocromil are alternatives for patients with mild disease)	Corticosteroid skin creams and ointments (see earlier article)	Consider need for standby adrenaline (refer to allergist)
Short course prednisolone (eg, prednisolone 20 mg/day for 5 days, peak season)	*Never* use corticosteroid eye drops without advice/supervision of ophthalmologist	Consider adding regular long acting inhaled bronchodilator (or theophylline tablets)	Antibiotics for exacerbations	
For severe hayfever refer to allergist for consideration for immunotherapy		Prednisolone tablets once daily in morning in lowest possible dose. Courses may be required at any time for exacerbations	Referral to dermatologist for consideration of skin wraps, behavioural therapy, and (rarely) prednisolone tablets	Consider immunotherapy (in allergy to bee or wasp venom)—refer to allergist

Avoidance measures for house dust mites should focus mainly on the bedroom. The room should be ventilated regularly; mattresses, pillows, and duvets should be encased in mite proof allergen covers (which may be left in place for up to six months) with the usual bed covers for mattress, pillows, and duvet put on over the top. Patients should be advised to launder this bedding every 1-2 weeks at 60°C. Vacuum cleaners with an adequate filter to remove house dust mite allergen and prevent dissemination through the vacuum exhaust have been recommended by the British Allergy Foundation. Removal of the bedroom carpet (where possible) is important. Soft toys should be reduced to a minimum and be washable; they may be placed regularly in a freezer to kill the mites. Even when these measures are applied conscientiously improvement may take 3-6 months.

When pet allergy is diagnosed, the offending animal (and if possible all furry animals) should be excluded from the home. Psychosocial considerations may mean that the best that can be achieved is confining the animal outside or in the kitchen, with a recommendation not to replace an animal. Again, advice to remove the bedroom carpet should be given. Some studies have shown that washing a cat weekly (cat allergens are present on the fur and are extremely water soluble) may reduce allergen load when combined with removal of the bedroom carpet. Even if the pet is removed, vigorous cleaning for 3-6 months afterwards is required to minimise pet allergen concentrations in the home.

It is unlikely that patients with summer hay fever will be able to avoid pollens. The best aim should be control of symptoms with topical corticosteroids and antihistamines so that the patient may lead as normal a life as possible. Patients with severe hay fever, however, should keep windows shut (cars and buildings); wear glasses or sunglasses; avoid grassy spaces, especially in the evening, when pollen counts are highest; fit a pollen filter to the car; and consider a holiday by the sea or abroad at peak times.

The practice nurse routinely provides individualised written instructions for asthmatic patients—about drug treatment, need for peak flow monitoring, inhaler technique, etc. He or she may also advise on allergen avoidance and environmental

Bed covers recommended by manufacturer as mite proof*

Alprotec Allergen Exclusion System—Advanced Allergy Technologies (0161 903 9293)
Allerayde Perfect Allergy Control—Allerayde (01636 613444)
Jonelle Zipped Mattress Liner—John Lewis Partnership (contact local branches)
Sandra Actifresh PVC Mattress cover—The Linen Cupboard (0171 629 4062)
Medivac Anti-Allergic Bedding—Medivac Health Care Products (01625 539401)
Medibed Supreme Mattress Barrier Protector—Medibed (01282 839700)
Health Beds—Sarah Street, Rotherham, South Yorkshire S61 1EF (01709 561937)
*"Breatheable" covers let water vapour through and are more comfortable than plastic

Vacuum cleaners recommended by British Allergy Foundation

- Hoover Pure Power Range (U3141, U3142 (1400S class) U3150 U3250 (1500S class), Hoover European Appliance Group, Pentrebach, Merthyr Tydfil CF48 4TU (tel: 01685 721222)
- HVR 200P Vacuum Cleaner (Cylinder), Neumatic International Limited, Millfield Road, Chard, Somerset TA20 2GB (tel: 01460 68480)
- Vorwerk VK121ET 340, Vorwerk UK, Ashville Way, Wokingham, Berkshire RG41 2PL (tel: 0118 979 4878)
- Sebo Automatic XI Vacuum Cleaner/Upright Airbelt C1 Cylinder, Sebo UK, Merlin Centre, Lancaster Road, High Wycombe, Buckinghamshire HP12 3QL (tel: 01494 465533)

control measures. The nurse may also advise patients with rhinitis how to use nasal sprays: blow the nose; tilt head so the chin is resting on the chest; hold the spray bottle upright and place nozzle just inside one nostril; apply one or two sprays as prescribed; repeat with the other nostril.

Occasionally corticosteroid nasal drops may be required, particularly for rhinosinusitis. These should be taken in the "head upside down position," best achieved by lying on your back on a bed, tilting your head right over the edge of the bed, applying drops to both nostrils and waiting for two minutes before getting up.

A Medic Alert bracelet or necklace (with an inscription that alerts other doctors to the possible cause of any future reaction) is very valuable for people at risk of anaphylaxis—for example, in response to penicillin, stinging insects, foods, or latex—and for patients with asthma who have sensitivity to aspirin. The practice nurse may teach patients how to use syringes of injectable adrenaline (epinephrine)—usually this will follow recommendation by an allergy specialist.

General practitioners can obtain a list of NHS allergy clinics from the British Society for Allergy and Clinical Immunology.

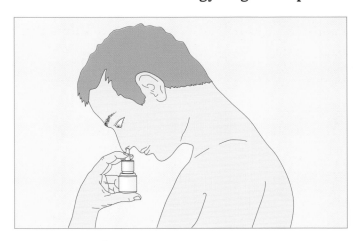

How to use a nasal spray

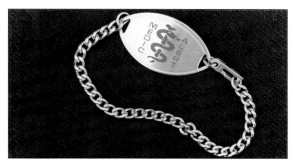

Medic Alert bracelet: important for patients at risk of anaphylaxis

The way forward

Many primary care practices already benefit from clinics devoted to the management of asthma, one of the common diseases frequently associated with allergy. Taking an allergy history with or without skin prick tests may enhance the effectiveness of asthma care. Skin testing with a limited range of reagents in general practice is both practicable and desirable. The recognition of the importance of rhinitis and the role of allergy in rhinitis and eczema will also enhance the management of atopic patients in general practice. Food allergy and occupational allergy should be considered; if such allergies are present, the patient should be referred to a specialist. The logical person to deliver allergen avoidance advice is the practice nurse, supported by the primary care doctor, and, where necessary, the local allergy service, whether provided by an NHS based specialist allergist or an organ-based specialist with training in allergy. Further studies are currently in progress to define those patients who are most likely to respond to allergen avoidance measures. Specialist referral may be needed too. The allergist may also effectively evaluate the role of allergy in patients presenting with non-specific symptoms—for example, the so-called multiple chemical sensitivity syndrome.

The Medic Alert Foundation provided the picture of the Medic Alert bracelet.

Useful organisations
- British Society for Allergy and Clinical Immunology, 66 Weston Park, Thames Ditton, Surrey KT7 0HL (tel: 0181 398 9240)
- British Allergy Foundation, Deepdene House, 30 Bellegrove Road, Welling, Kent DA16 3BY (patients' helpline: 0181 303 8583)
- National Asthma Campaign, Providence House, Providence Place, London N1 0NT (tel: 0171 226 2260)
- Anaphylaxis Campaign, PO Box 149, Fleet, Hampshire GU13 9XU (tel: 01252 542029; fax: 01252 377140)
- Medic Alert Foundation, 17 Bridge Wharf, 156 Caledonian Road, London N1 9UU (tel: 0171 833 3034; fax: 0171 713 5653)
- National Asthma and Respiratory Training Centre, The Athenaeum, 10 Church Street, Warwick CV34 4AB (tel: 01926 493313; fax: 01926 493224; email: enquiries@nartc.org.uk)

When to refer patients for specialist allergy advice
- For investigation and management of anaphylaxis
- If the diagnosis of allergy is in doubt—for example, discordance between the clinical history and the results of skin prick testing or the radioallergosorbent test
- If food allergy is suspected (for assessment and expert dietetic input)
- If occupational allergy is suspected
- In cases of urticaria in which an allergic aetiology is suspected
- For consideration for immunotherapy (in cases of severe hay fever, allergy to venom from stinging insects)
- To exclude allergy as a cause of non-specific illness

Further reading
- Sibbald B, Barnes G, Durham SR. Skin prick testing in general practice: a pilot study. *J Adv Nurs* 1997;26:537-42
- The British guidelines on asthma management 1995. Review and position statement. *Thorax* 1997;52(suppl 1)
- Lund V on behalf of the International Rhinitis Management Working Group. International consensus report on the diagnosis and management of rhinitis. *Allergy* 1994;49(suppl 19):1-34

Index

Index